UNDERSTANDING NEUROLOGIC DISEASE

UNDERSTANDING NEUROLOGIC DISEASE

A Textbook
for Therapists

John H. Warfel, Ph.D.
and
Reinhold E. Schlagenhauff, M.D.

State University of New York at Buffalo
School of Medicine

Urban & Schwarzenberg • Baltimore-Munich 1980

Urban & Schwarzenberg, Inc.
7 E. Redwood Street
Baltimore, Maryland 21202
USA

Urban & Schwarzenberg
Pettenkoferstrasse 18
D-8000 München 2
GERMANY

Library of Congress Cataloging in Publication Data

Warfel, John H.
  Understanding neurologic disease.

  Includes bibliographical references and index.
  1. Nervous system—Diseases.   2. Physical therapists.
  I. Schlagenhauff, Reinhold E., joint author.   II. Title. [DNLM:
  1. Nervous system diseases—Diagnosis.   2. Nervous system diseases—Therapy.   3. Occupational therapy.   4. Physical therapy.
  WL100.3 W274u]
  RC346.W29   616.8   79–28455
  ISBN 0–8067–2131–6

ISBN 0–8067–2131–6   (Baltimore)
ISBN 3–541–72131–6   (Munich)

Printed in the United States of America

CONTENTS

DEDICATION

To our wives, Marjorie Wolfe Warfel and Erika Krimm Schlagenhauff and to therapy students everywhere.

PREFACE

This book is the result of material presented to the Physical and Occupational Therapy students at SUNY, Buffalo in the neurology portion of their course in Neurosciences. It was originally made available as a loose-leaf manual with two objectives in mind: first, to facilitate and minimize note taking by the student; second, to serve as a handy reference source during the student's clinical affiliation and later professional career.

The material presented in the lectures and herein has been selected on the basis of many years experience we have had in teaching neuroanatomy and neurology to therapy students. It is designed to give the student an understanding of the various neurologic problems which are likely to be encountered in working with the physically handicapped. This should enable the student to recognize the clinical signs and symptoms of neurologic diseases as they frequently occur, to better appreciate the medical management of the problem after the diagnosis is established with the possibility of offering a prognosis.

Through discussion with practicing therapists and former students the authors have been made aware of the fact that many educational institutions which offer programs in Physical and Occupational Therapy are not fortunate enough to have available the services of a clinical neurologist on their faculties or the facilities for patient demonstrations to the students during their training prior to clinical affiliation.

Accordingly, the third objective of our efforts is to make available to teachers and students alike that clinical approach which may be lacking in their pre-clinical training.

Over the years there has been a demand on therapists for an increased knowledge of neurologic disease. Our efforts here are to present this material in a basic manner so that the student of neurology may acquire this knowledge without the burden of the minutiae of details. Hence, this work is not meant to be a complete treatise on clinical neurology or to offer a means of therapeutic management. For more detailed information the reader is advised to consult comprehensive textbooks of neurology and the appropriate works on rehabilitation.

J.H.W.
R.E.S.

UNDERSTANDING
NEUROLOGIC
DISEASE

Chapter 1

NEURODIAGNOSTIC PRINCIPLES

Neurology is the science of diseases affecting the brain and spinal cord, the peripheral nerves, and the autonomic division of the nervous system. A background of neuroanatomy is required to enable the student to locate the site of the lesion in the conditions discussed in the following chapters.

NEUROLOGIC EXAMINATION

Before starting the interview the neurologist tries to put the patient completely at ease. The physician first takes a good *history*, which may require 30 to 45 minutes, but this is time well spent. *In many cases the diagnosis may be arrived at by a good historical evaluation.*

Different types of neurologic diseases present different profiles. If the symptoms are intermittently present, cardiovascular problems may be suspected. Symptoms usually subside after relatively minor trauma and increase in severity in cases of tumors.

Forgetfulness, episodes of unconsciousness and behavior problems may require a relative or friend to accompany the patient in order to supply additional important information. It is also valuable to know whether the patient is left-handed, right-handed or ambidexterous (to determine the dominant cerebral hemisphere).

Neurologic problems frequently occur in association with other medical diseases, complicating these disorders and their treatment. For example, hypertension may cause cerebral involvement (stroke), and diabetes mellitus may involve the brain, peripheral nerves and autonomic nervous system. Metabolic disorders usually involve the central nervous system diffusely and slightly more than peripheral nerves. Cancer elsewhere in the body may produce metastatic tumors in the central nervous system. Infectious diseases with high fever may cause stupor, confusion, uncooperative behavior and even unconsciousness. Fainting episodes can occur in severe anemia.

The above are just a few examples of medical diseases that can affect the nervous system; therefore, the neurologic history should always include a careful medical history going back to the patient's birth and early life. A family history may be important for inherited types of disorders, which frequently occur (autosomal, sex-linked, dominant or recessive). During the interview the patient is carefully observed in regard to behavior, mannerism, mood changes and delusions.

The neurologic examination is done to determine:

- The presence or absence of a neurologic disorder.
- The location, size and type of a lesion.
- The degree to which the unaffected or normal
  parts may be used for rehabilitation.

The examination starts with the higher functions—that is, those of the cerebrum, cranial nerves, and cerebellum. The neurologist then checks in turn the motor system, sensory system, and reflexes. Finally, if necessary, a number of neurodiagnostic tests are available for more precise diagnosis.

A. THE HIGHER FUNCTIONS

1. Cerebrum

a) **Behavior,** manner of dress, gestures and cooperation
   are observed.

b) The level of consciousness is evaluated. It is important to observe whether the patient is alert, attentive, drowsy or stuporous. The examiner tries to find out whether the patient is on medication.

c) Intellectual performance is next evaluated, based on educational, economic and geographical background. An IQ level below 70 indicates mental retardation.

d) Memory is evaluated. For example, in cerebral arteriosclerosis recent memory is impaired first. It is important to check orientation as to time (date, month, year), place and person. The patient should know where he is and remember his name.

e) Emotional states frequently influence neurologic complaints. For example, the patient may be depressed, euphoric or reveal hostility or negativism.

f) Thought processes are carefully observed. The patient may be preoccupied with his or her condition. He may reveal a repetition of complaints (perseveration). He or she may be overimaginative or have bizzare ideas of persecution. Delusions or hallucinations may occur during the examination. It is also very important to establish whether or not the patient has insight into his condition.

To judge these cerebral functions it is important to know that frontal lobe functions involve behavior, personality, intellectual performance, initiative and drive. The process by which emotional problems become transformed into physical symptoms (motor or sensory) is called *conversion.* Specific cerebral functions are localized in certain areas of the brain:

VISUAL—occipital cortex

AUDITORY—temporal cortex

TACTILE—parietal cortex
(Including relationship of body parts to each other)

MOTOR—precentral gyrus

SENSORY—postcentral gyrus

The student needs to understand the terms for specific impairments and loss of cerebral function:

Paralysis. The complete loss of voluntary movement in a muscle through injury or disease of its nerve supply.

Paresis. Partial weakness or incomplete paralysis.

Apraxia. The incapacity to execute purposeful or skillful movements.

Agnosia. The loss of ability to recognize the importance of sensory stimuli. It corresponds to the different senses and is recognized as auditory, visual, olfactory, gustatory or tactile.

Aphasia. The loss of expression by speech, writing or gestures, or of comprehension of spoken or written language. It may be *expressive* and located in the posterior inferior frontal lobe (Broca's area), or *receptive*, located in the upper temporal lobe (Wernicke's area). These regions are frequently affected in strokes or brain tumors located in the dominant hemisphere. If the expressive aphasia has been complete, the first word usually to come back after speech loss is "no." (The patient has to re-learn his entire vocabulary as in childhood.)

After testing the general cerebral functions and observing specific cerebral manifestations, the neurologist next examines the cranial nerves.

2. Cranial Nerves

By convention there are 12 pairs of cranial nerves.

Olfactory nerve (I)

Optic nerve (II)

Oculomotor nerve (III)

Trochlear nerve (IV)

Abducens nerve (VI)

Trigeminal nerve (V)

Facial nerve (VII)

Vestibulocochlear nerve (VIII)

Glossopharyngeal nerve (IX)

Vagus nerve (X)

Accessory nerve (XI)

Hypoglossal nerve (XII)

Olfactory nerve (I)

First the nasal passageways are checked to determine that they are open and not obstructed. Then each nostril should be tested separately with agents such as perfume, soap, or tobacco (with the patient's eyes closed). The inability to smell on one side may be indicative of trauma and injury to the cribriform plate of the ethmoid bone, causing rupture of olfactory fibers. It may also suggest a brain tumor compressing the olfactory nerve (olfactory groove meningioma). Absence of the sense of smell on both sides is relatively rare and usually occurs in very severe trauma or on a psychogenic basis.

Optic nerve (II)

The examination is done with an ophthalmoscope, and the fundus, including the optic disks, are carefully evaluated. The optic disk is swollen in cases of brain tumor (disk edema or papilledema). Atrophy of the optic disk occurs with syphilitic involvement of the central nervous system. In multiple sclerosis (MS) the temporal half of the optic disk is pale, while the nasal half remains normal.

Occasionally hemorrhages can be seen on the fundus (central or peripheral), especially with increased intracranial pressure. The retinal veins and their branches are crossed by arteries. Compression of the veins in pronounced hypertension results in "arterio-venous nicking" (Fig. 1).

There are several degrees of A-V nicking that can be recognized, depending on the severity of the elevated blood pressure.

Then the visual fields are tested for defects. Tunnel (gun-barrel) vision occurs mainly in psychogenic disorders (occasionally in tertiary syphilis).

Oculomotor nerve (III). ⎫
Trochlear nerve (IV). ⎬ These nerves supply the musculature for eye movements.
Abducens nerve (VI). ⎭

The oculomotor nerve also supplies the muscles which constrict the pupils (parasympathetic fibers) and elevate the eyelids. The range of eye movement is checked by asking the patient to follow the movement of the examiner's finger while the finger is moved in several directions of gaze.

If the *oculomotor nerve* is completely involved the patient will not be able to look up, down or medially with the affected eye.

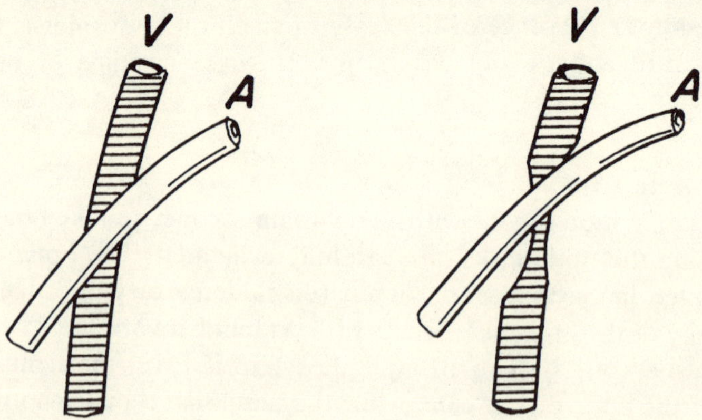

Figure 1.   Arterio-venous nicking. Left-hand figure shows normal A-V crossing; right-hand figure shows compression of underlying vein by hypertensive artery.

There will also be ptosis (drooping) of the eyelid and dilation of the pupil.

If the *trochlear nerve* is involved, the patient is unable to look downward in lateral gaze. If the *abducens nerve* is affected the patient is unable to look laterally on the involved side.

In any of these conditions the patient may complain of double vision. During the examination the eyes are also checked for nystagmus (oscillatory movements of the eyeballs) and pupillary size.

The diameter of the pupils, their shape and equality are also noted. The pupillary reaction to light flashes and accommodation is tested (frequently impaired in neuro-syphilis and known as Argyll Robertson pupil).

In general the pupils are larger in younger persons and become smaller and less responsive to light in the elderly population. Both direct and consensual (the similar reaction of both pupils to a stimulus applied to only one) pupillary reflexes are observed.

Since the abducens nerve is rather long within the cranial cavity, as compared to the other cranial nerves, it is frequently affected as a false localizing sign and cannot always be used for localizing purposes. For example, this nerve is often involved in cerebral tumors with increased intracranial pressure.

***Trigeminal nerve* (V)**

The masseter and temporalis muscles are examined first by palpating them when the jaws are clenched together. The examiner looks for any deviation of the jaw when the mouth is open. Because of the sensory innervation, the skin of the face is checked for several modalities such as touch, pinprick and temperature. The patient should be able to feel cotton as well as a needle touching the forehead and cheeks.

Differences in the response to touch and pinprick from one side to the other are noted. The patient should have his eyes closed during the procedure.

The corneal reflex is tested by touching the cornea with a wisp of cotton. This reflex should be elicited equally on both sides and is very helpful in determining the degree of a comatose state.

The jaw jerk is tested by tapping the middle of the chin with a reflex hammer while the patient's mouth is slightly open. Normally a slight closing movement of the jaw is observed; this can be exaggerated in cases of pyramidal tract diseases.

Facial nerve (VII)

Sensory fibers supply the anterior two-thirds of the tongue for taste. With the eyes closed and the tongue protruded, the patient should be checked for sensation to sweet, sour, salty and bitter agents. This is usually done on one side and then the other.

The motor distribution is to the muscles of facial expression. The patient is asked to wrinkle his forehead, to close his eyes and to open his mouth. In *peripheral* seventh nerve involvement (Bell's palsy) all motor branches are affected. In *upper motor neuron* involvement, because of the bilateral cortical representation, only the lower part of the face is affected.

Vestibulocochlear nerve (VIII)

This nerve is divided into two portions, vestibular and cochlear. For the cochlear nerve a tuning fork (256 cycles) is used to check air and bone conduction. The fork is placed on the forehead to test hearing on the right and left (Weber's test).

When bone versus air conduction is tested the fork is usually placed over the mastoid process (Rinne's test). Normally, bone conduction stops before air conduction because bone is not as good a sound conductor as air. The vestibular portion of the nerve is checked for abnormal rapid (oscillatory) eye movements indicative of nystagmus.

The patient is also asked to walk on a straight line with his eyes closed; there should be no deviation to either side.

Glossopharyngeal nerve (IX)

A tongue blade is used, and while the patient says "ah" the uvula should move straight upward (there should be no major post-surgical scar formation in the faucial isthmus). The gag reflex is checked for sensory function.

Vagus nerve (X)

The normal function of this nerve is revealed by the patient's ability to swallow and to speak without hoarseness. Occasionally the vocal cords have to be inspected to look for asymmetrical movements. The autonomic functions of the nerve are evaluated during the general physical examination. In vagus nerve palsy there will be tachycardia (accelerated heart rate).

Accessory nerve (XI)

The functions of the trapezius and sternocleidomastoid muscles are tested on both sides by having the patient shrug his shoulders one at a time and by turning his head to either side.

Hypoglossal nerve (XII)

The patient is asked to stick out his tongue; any lateral deviation of the tongue is noted. The examiner looks for atrophy or tremor. The strength of the tongue musculature can be tested by having the patient move the tongue from side to side against the cheeks.

Occasionally fasciculations of the tongue can be observed while the tongue is at rest on the floor of the mouth. Pathologically, the tongue, when protruded, deviates to the side of the nerve lesion.

3. Cerebellum

The testing of cerebellar functions begins by asking the patient to place a finger on his nose (eyes closed) or on the finger of the examiner (eyes open). Besides the finger-nose test one can also observe the heel-knee test, in which the patient is asked to run the heel of one foot down the shin of the opposite leg.

Next, the ability to perform rapid and alternate movements is evaluated. With cerebellar lesions unsteadiness (ataxia) is noted; the patient will be unable to walk by placing one foot in front of the other (tandem gait). After this the Romberg sign is looked for; in this test the patient stands with his feet together and his arms out in front with his eyes closed. If the Romberg test is positive the patient may fall to either side, forwards or backwards. *Intention tremor* (as in the finger-nose test) is often observed; in this condition the tremor develops at the end of execution of a purposeful act. In testing for "rebound phenomena," the patient's arm is extended with the forearm flexed in a vertical position. The examiner tries to pull the forearm away from the patient against resistance. If the forearm is suddenly released, normally the hand will not strike the patient's face or shoulder as it may do in cerebellar disease.

Having checked the higher neurological functions, the neurologist examines the motor and sensory systems.

B. THE MOTOR SYSTEM

Examination of the motor mechanisms begins by comparing the muscles of the upper and lower extremities on one side with those of the opposite side for equality of size (taking into consideration minor differences due to cerebral dominance). A tape measure can be used to compare corresponding parts.

Percussion of the tongue or of the thenar eminence may reveal myotonic responses (muscle contraction with slow relaxation). While examining the muscles of each extremity the examiner looks for wasting (atrophy) or spontaneous muscle movement such as fasciculations or tremor of the fingers. Fasciculations can frequently be observed with muscle wasting, due to lower motor neuron involvement. The tone of the musculature is evaluated and this may be found to be normal, decreased or increased.

Usually, in the acute phase of a stroke, a decreased tone of the paralyzed limb is seen for approximately five to seven days;

thereafter the tone is usually increased to "jackknife" spasticity in cases of pyramidal tract disease. In extrapyramidal tract disease the tone may be increased, but this increased tone is of the "cogwheel" type.

In peripheral nerve lesions or myopathies the muscle tone is usually decreased. Muscle strength is tested by the examiner, comparing corresponding muscles on each side. The involved nerves, their motor distribution and the clinical signs are summarized in Table 1.

C. THE SENSORY SYSTEM

The examiner first establishes that the patient is able to perceive the sensation being tested and then compares both sides of the body and the extremities. (This cannot be accomplished in confused mental states.) In all sensory tests the patient should keep the eyes closed. Touch, pain and temperature are tested on various areas of the skin. For touch a piece of cotton or the finger is used; for pain a pin. Temperature is tested by using cold and warm water in test tubes. A tuning fork is used to test vibratory sense.

Touching the upper or lower extremities simultaneously on both sides is a test for checking a lesion in the parietal lobe. In this type of lesion the contralateral side is neglected (extinction phenomenon). Stimulation of the palm of the hand in adults may result in a "grasp reflex" (normally present in early infancy) which is seen in frontal lobe lesions.

D. REFLEXES

After the sensory examination, the patient is tested for deep tendon reflexes, superficial reflexes, and pathological reflexes.

1. Deep Tendon Reflexes

These are compared on both sides of the body. The *biceps reflex* (C5–C6) is tested by hitting the biceps tendon with the reflex hammer; normally a contraction of the biceps muscle will result. The *brachioradialis reflex* (C5–C6) is tested by hitting the styloid process of the radius, resulting in forearm flexion and pronation. The *triceps brachii* (C7–C8) is tested by tapping the triceps tendon above the olecranon process, resulting in extension of the forearm.

The most important deep tendon reflex is probably the *patellar reflex* (L2–L3–L4), which is elicited by tapping the patellar tendon, resulting in extension of the leg at the knee joint. The *Achilles tendon* reflex (S1–S2) represents the longest reflex arc in the body and is frequently affected by metabolic or hormonal disorders. Normally, tapping the tendon results in plantar flexion of the foot. Frequently in the elderly, the Achilles tendon reflex is diminished or absent. An increased duration of this reflex is seen in hypothyroidism or Parkinsonism, where the relaxation phase of the reflex is prolonged.

In severe pyramidal tract disease *ankle clonus* often occurs; this is manifested by a sustained or unsustained rapid, alternating dorsi- and plantar flexion of the foot. The clonus can be elicited by briskly dorsi-flexing the foot with mild pressure.

2. Superficial Reflexes

These are tested by lightly stroking the skin without scratching it. The *abdominal reflexes* (T8–T12) are important. The upper abdominal reflex will move the umbilicus upward toward the area being stroked; the lower abdominal muscles will reflexly move the umbilicus downward. These reflexes are frequently absent in pyramidal tract diseases.

In the male patient the cremasteric reflex (T12–L1) is tested by stimulating the inside of the thigh. A normal response is elevation of the scrotum on the ipsilateral side.

Stroking the plantar part of the foot (S1–S2) normally results in flexion of the toes. Finally, the gluteal reflex (L4–S3) is tested by stroking the area around the anus, which will elicit tension of the skin in the gluteal area.

Table 1.

Nerves	Motor Distribution	Clinical Signs
Brachial Plexus		
1. Long thoracic	Serratus anterior	"Winged scapula"
2. Thoracodorsal	Latissimus dorsi	Loss of arm adduction and extension
3. Dorsal scapular	Rhomboids; levator scapulae	Loss of scapular adduction and elevation
4. Suprascapular	Supraspinatus Infraspinatus	Weakened lateral rotation of humerus
5. Subscapular	Subscapularis Teres major	Weakened medial rotation of humerus
6. Radial	All extensors of arm and forearm	"Wrist drop"
7. Axillary	Deltoid Teres minor	Loss of arm abduction; weakened lateral rotation of humerus
8. Musculocutaneous	Coracobrachialis Brachialis Biceps brachii	Loss of forearm flexion and supination
9. Median	Flexors of hand and digits; opponens pollicis	"Ape hand" deformity; weakened grip; loss of thumb opposition
10. Ulnar	Flexor of hand and digits; adductor pollicis	"Claw hand" deformity; weakened grip; loss of thumb adduction.
Lumbosacral Plexus		
1. Femoral	Iliopsoas; quadriceps femoris	Loss of thigh flexion, leg extension
2. Obturator	Adductors of thigh	Weakened or loss of thigh adduction
3. Sciatic	Hamstrings; all musculature below the knee	Loss of leg flexion; paralysis of all muscles of leg and foot
a. Common peroneal	Dorsiflexors of foot	"Foot drop"; "steppage gait"; loss of eversion
b. Tibial	Gastrocnemius; soleus; deep plantar flexors of foot	Loss of plantar flexion and inversion of foot

3. Pathological Reflexes

These are seen in pyramidal tract diseases and are as follows:

Babinski   This is the most important reflex and is elicited by stimulating the lateral aspect of the sole of the foot. In pyramidal tract diseases dorsi-flexion of the big toe occurs as well as fanning of the other toes. It should be remembered that this reflex is normal in infants up to age 16 months, after which time it disappears.

Chaddock   Gives the same type of response as the Babinski phenomenon. For this reflex, however, the lateral aspect of the foot beneath and around the lateral malleolus is stimulated.

Oppenheim   Extension of the great toe will result from stimulation of the antero-medial aspect of the leg (rubbing the shin).

Gordon   This reflex, elicited by squeezing the calf musculature, produces extension and fanning as described for the Babinski phenomenon.

Rossolimo   Plantar flexion of the toes occurs when the plantar surface of the toes is tapped.

Mendel-Bechterew   Hitting the foot above the area of the cuboid bone results in plantar flexion of the toes in pyramidal tract disease.

E. NEURODIAGNOSTIC TESTS

These tests described below are done for detailed examination, especially of the central nervous system, and require sophisticated equipment operated by skilled technicians. The results are interpreted by the neurologist.

1. X-Rays (Skull, Neck and other parts of body)

Antero-posterior (A-P) and lateral views are taken. In adults we look for calcification of the pineal gland, which occurs after the age of 16, and try to determine whether it is in midline or deviated. A shift of more than 2 mm. to either side is pathologic.

The radiologist determines whether any fracture lines can be detected and looks for abnormal intracerebral calcifications (as with toxoplasmosis and tuberous sclerosis). Frontal, maxillary and ethmoidal sinus involvement, in cases of sinusitis, is checked.

Bony changes in the mastoid process or in the temporal region, due to infectious processes, are looked for. The size of the sella turcica, which is enlarged in cases of pituitary tumors, is determined. The bony structures of the sella may be eroded or atrophic in cases of chronic increased intracranial pressure.

In children this may cause widening of the bony sutures. Brain swelling may cause indentation of the bone by the swollen gyri (prominent convolutional markings) and change the normally rather smooth X-ray appearance of the inner table of the skull.

A space-occupying lesion in the area of the foramen magnum may widen the foramen.

In all cases of head injury X-rays of the cervical vertebrae (A-P, lateral and oblique) should be taken because of frequent simultaneous damage in this region.

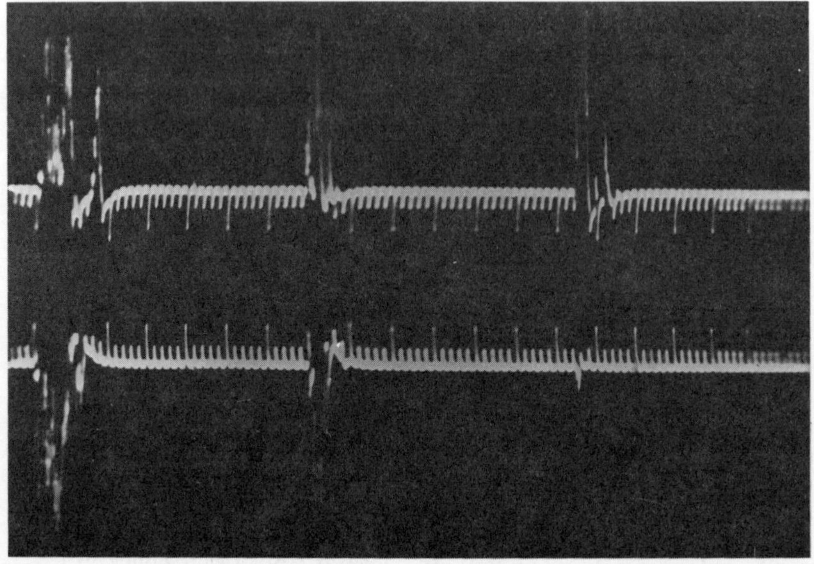

Figure 2.   Echoencephalogram with midline ventricular system. Posterior third ventricle measures 6 mm in diameter in this 45-year-old man with mild central and cortical cerebral atrophy. (Diameter of head 13.3 cm; large markings 1 cm, small markings 2 mm.)

In cases of peripheral nerve injuries X-rays of the involved bony structures of the extremities may be necessary (to determine wrist abnormalities in carpal tunnel syndrome; bony changes at the medial epicondyle of the humerus in ulnar nerve involvement, etc.).

2. Ultrasonography

A-mode Echoencephalography (Fig. 2) has been widely used to determine the shift of the midline structures (represented by the third ventricle). In this test an ultrasonic device that produces sound frequencies of 2.25 MHz is used. The ultrasonic waves will hit the third ventricle, the lateral ventricles and the opposite side of the skull.

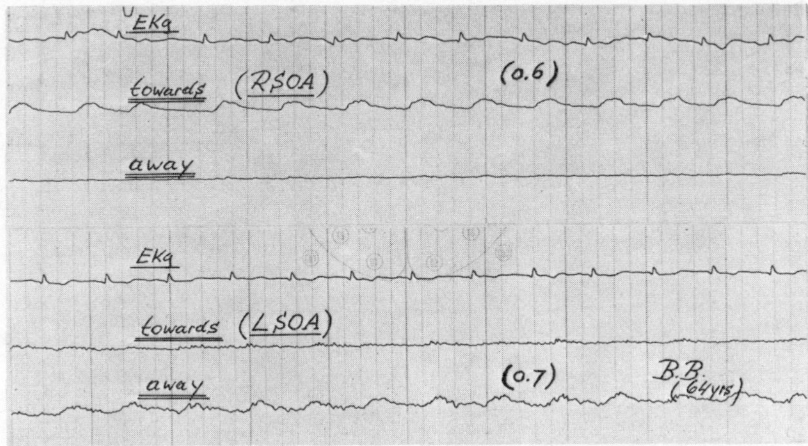

Figure 3.   Doppler Ultrasonogram of 64-year-old patient with left internal carotid artery occlusion. Bloodflow of the left supra-orbital artery is strongly reversed (lower part) as compared to the normal flow of the right supra-orbital artery (upper part).

A difference in acoustic impedance will give an interface which will send back an echo, and this will be recorded on the oscilloscope. Any shift of more than 2 mm. is pathologic. The procedure is benign, does not cause any harm to the brain and can be repeated frequently. Ultrasonography, as described here, is accurate in approximately 90% of the cases.

Echoencephalography can be used during craniotomy to find out the following about a tumor:

- Where it is closest to the surface.
- Its general shape.
- Its depth.

In this procedure a sterile probe has to be used.

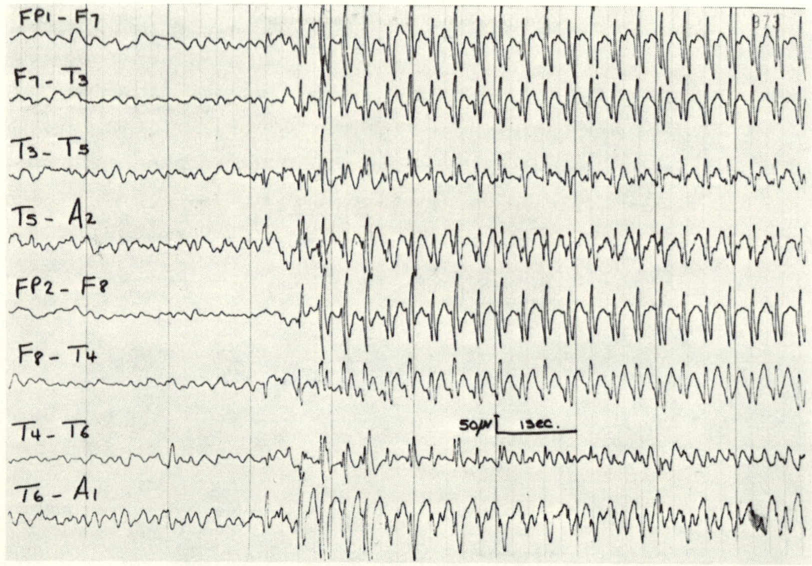

Figure 4.   Electroencephalogram of 12-year-old boy with minor and occasional major seizures. On left, fairly normal background rhythm, on right, bilateral synchronous and symmetrical spike and wave complexes at 3–4 cycles/second, maximal on frontal regions (consistent with cortico-reticular type of epileptiform disorder).

Doppler Ultrasonography

Doppler ultrasonic flowmeter studies are used in vascular insufficiencies to study hemodynamics. This test uses a 10 MHz device to detect the blood flow in arteries or veins (Fig. 3). The common carotid, supraorbital, vertebral, brachial, radial, femoral, popliteal and dorsalis pedis arteries can be checked. In severe stenosis or occlusion of the internal carotid artery at the area of the bifurcation, the blood flow in the supraorbital artery is commonly reversed.

3. Electroencephalography (EEG)

In this procedure the machine used is basically a polygraph (Fig. 4). Twenty-two electrodes are pasted on various parts of the patient's head according to generally accepted criteria (10–20 International System). The patient is usually recumbent and possibly slightly sedated in order to achieve sleep.

This device is mainly used to determine the electrical potentials of the cerebral cortex, whether or not epileptiform discharges are present, to localize destructive lesions and to determine whether "brain death" has occurred. In this last case (with maximal amplification) an isoelectric recording will result.

The output of the EEG is registered according to the different waves, as follows:

Waves	*Cycles/Second*
Alpha:	8 to 13
Beta:	14 to 26
Theta:	4 to 7
Delta:	1 to 3

Eight-, 10- or 16-channel machines are used for recording different combinations of electrodes. In the electroencephalogram the brain potentials are magnified one million to ten million times. Epileptic discharges will show up as a spike or sharp wave focus. Structural lesions may be demonstrated by a slow wave focus. Metabolic disturbances affecting the brain will result in an increase of delta and theta waves, mainly on the anterior areas, throughout the record.

In overnight sleep recording, dream states are reflected by rapid eye movements (REM), which can be recorded. These episodes usually occur several times throughout the night and last normally from eight to 10 minutes each.

4. Spinal Puncture

Spinal puncture is done to screen the spinal fluid. It is *contraindicated* in disk edema and extreme swelling of the brain in cases of tumors or hemorrhages. A spinal needle is placed into the

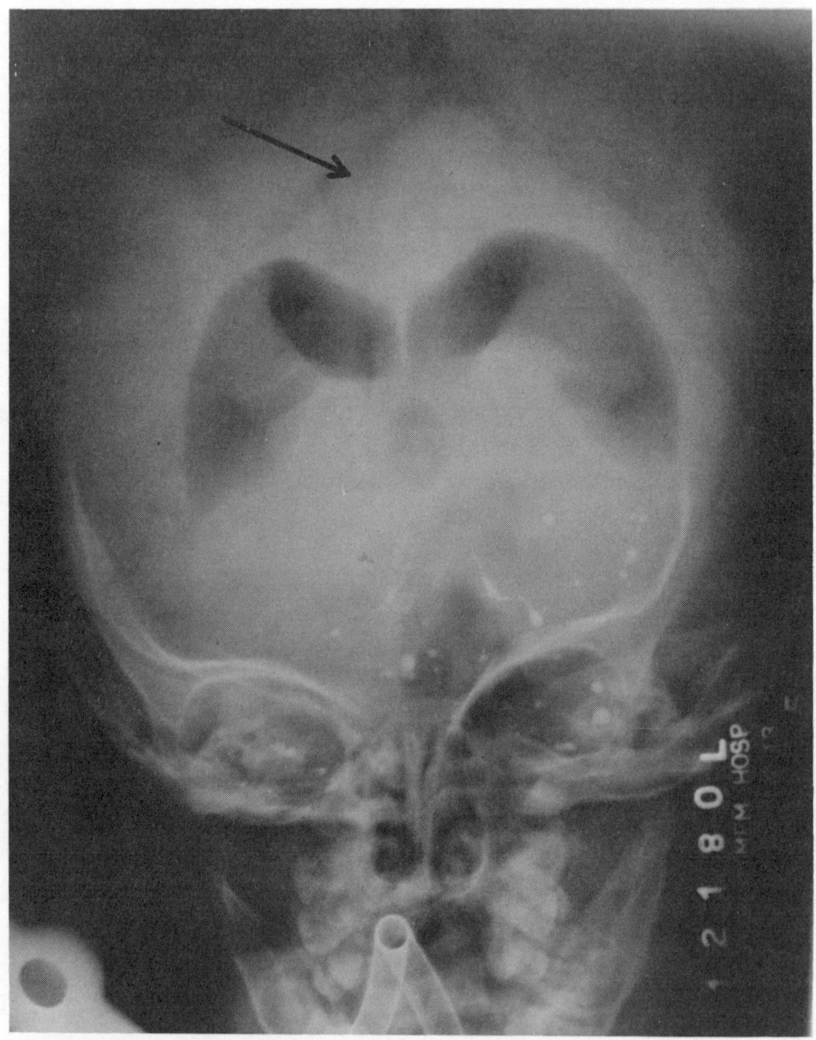

Figure 5.   Pneumoencephalogram of child (18 months) with marked and slightly asymmetrical dilation of lateral ventricles and third ventricle. Note enlarged head with separated sutures (arrow) in this case of hydrocephalus. (Courtesy of Dr. George Alker)

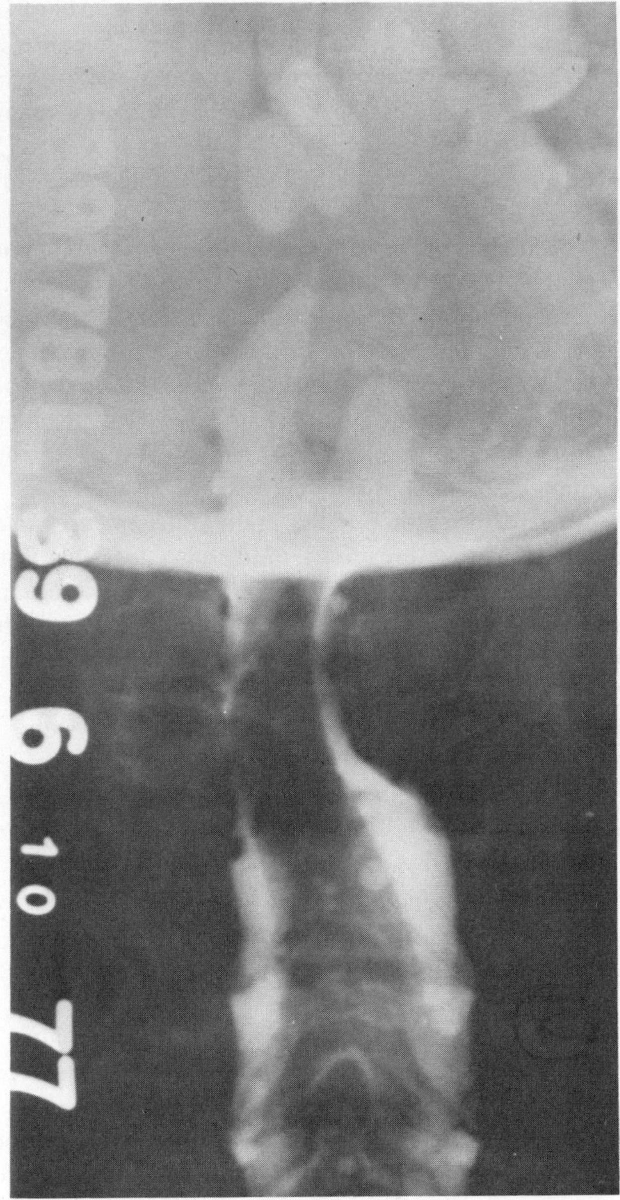

Figure 6.   Myelography in adult patient with neck tumor. The round-shaped and expanding lesion is compressing the cord and displacing the opaque material, which was placed into the spinal canal. (Courtesy of Dr. George Alker)

subarachnoid space in the lumbar region at the level of L3–L4. A manometer is used to check the spinal fluid pressure, which is normally between 100 and 170 mm. of water.

Space-occupying lesions may cause a pressure increase. After the pressure is determined, approximately 5–10 ml of fluid are removed for testing. The fluid removed should be clear and not contain any blood.

The cell count is determined and the protein content, which is normally between 30–40 mg%, is tested. The sugar level is evaluated and should be approximately 70% of the blood sugar level tested 30 minutes before.

Electrophoresis of the spinal fluid can be used to separate the alpha, beta and gamma globulins in cases of demyelinating diseases, luetic infections and space-occupying lesions. In these cases the gamma globulin is usually elevated.

Formerly, air studies of the brain (*Pneumoencephalography*) were done, but they are rarely used today. For this test, after a spinal tap is done, and some fluid removed, an equal amount of air is slowly injected (body upright); it tends to go into the lateral ventricles and also into the subarachnoid spaces surrounding the brain.

The size and position of the ventricular system are then checked by X-ray studies. The ventricular system may be dilated in cases of hydrocephalus and the sulci, on the convexity, may be widened in cases of cerebral atrophy (Fig. 5.) After this procedure the air is gradually resorbed and the patient requires 24 hours of bedrest. The test is *contraindicated* in cases of increased intracranial pressure (because of the possibility of cerebellar tonsillar herniation into the foramen magnum).

Frequently, a *Myelogram* will have to be performed, in cases of spinal cord lesions (disks, tumors, abscesses, injuries), to localize the exact position of the lesion before surgical exploration. After removal of a few milliliters of spinal fluid by spinal puncture, Metrizemide (Amipaque), which is a water-soluble radiographic contrast material, is injected into the subarachnoid space to pinpoint the level and outline the suspected abnormality (Fig. 6).

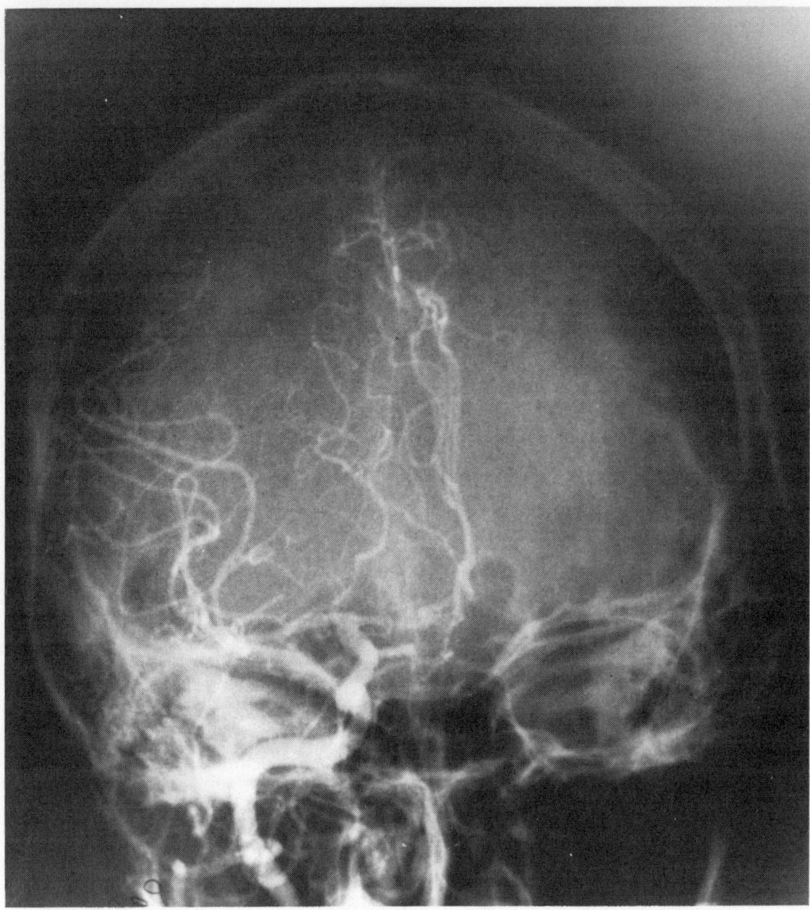

Figure 7.   Arteriogram of 55-year-old woman with malignant
and rapidly growing brain tumor of right hemisphere (glioblastoma multiforme). The arterial system, especially the anterior cerebral arteries, is displaced towards the left side.
(Courtesy of Dr. George Alker)

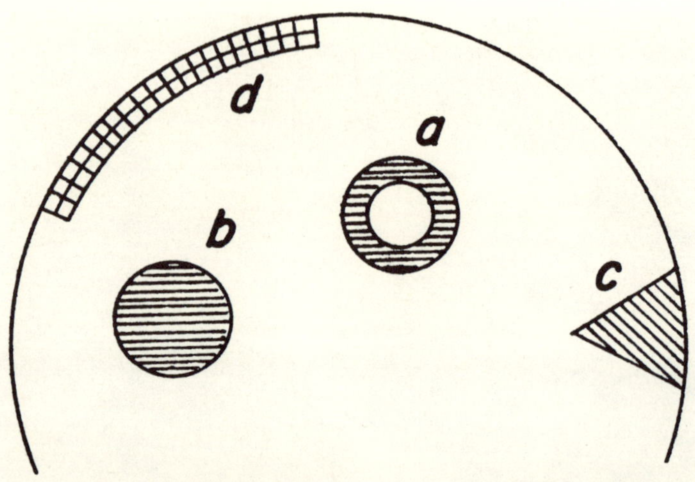

Figure 8.　Diagram of isotope brain scan and flow studies. (a) Abscess or cyst—a "doughnut shaped" uptake is found in cases of cerebral abscesses or cysts; (b) Tumor or hemorrhage—a circular pattern is usually indicative of a brain tumor or an intracerebral hemorrhage; (c) Infarction—triangular or wedge-shaped patterns are seen in cases of cerebral infarctions; (d) Sub- or epidural hematoma—uptake over the convexity of the brain is found in cases of subdural or epidural hematoma.

5. Cerebral Angiography

This test should be used only with great caution because complications occur frequently (emboli, thromboses, bleeding). Radiographic contrast material is injected into the arterial system by way of the brachial, carotid, vertebral or femoral arteries. Hypaque sodium visualizes the arteries of the brain. Usually, eight to 10 pictures are taken for demonstration of different intracranial vessels. Space-occupying lesions may cause displacement of blood vessels; highly vascularized tumors of the brain may show an increased uptake of the radiopaque material in the center. The test will also show blockage of an artery by an embolus. This invasive procedure is usually done only if there are fairly strong indications for surgical intervention (Fig. 7).

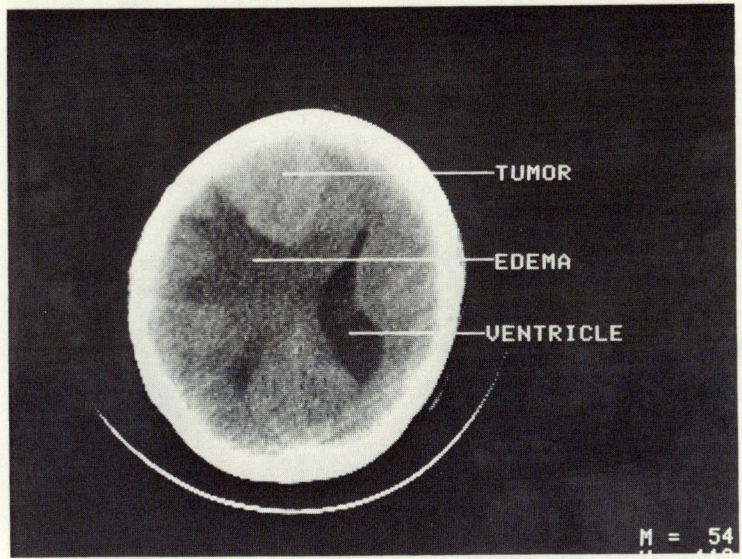

Figure 9.   CT-scan of 46-year-old woman with frontal space-occupying lesion (Meningioma). Considerable cerebral edema surrounds the tumor (increased density). The left lateral ventricle is compressed and slightly displaced. (Courtesy Dr. George Alker)

6. Isotope Brain Scan and Flow Studies

Radioactive material is injected into the venous system; Technetium 99M is generally used. The procedure is important in localizing brain tumors and cerebral infarctions (for the latter, after a latency period of seven to nine days). Uptake of the radioactive material is probably due to increased vascularity in the areas involved (Fig. 8).

7. CT-Scan

Computerized Axial Tomography (CT-Scan) (Fig. 9) is a computerized X-ray technique applied to the structures of the brain and was developed by Hounsfield in England. It is a non-invasive technique which makes tumor detection easier and, depending upon the equipment, takes only two to 15 minutes for an adequate picture of the brain structures. *Increased densities* are found with space-occupying lesions and *decreased densities* are found in cerebral vascular accidents (after 48–72 hours).

The CT-scan, which can also be used for the detection of focal or generalized atrophy, hydrocephalus, A-V malformations and cerebral cysts, has largely replaced pneumoencephalography and, to some extent, cerebral arteriography and isotope brain scanning.

CT-scan has also been applied to the area of the spinal cord to localize compressive lesions. Although the techniques in spinal cord lesions are not as yet firmly established, promising studies are continuing. CT equipment and the procedure are both expensive.

8. Electroneuromyography

Electroneuromyography (EMG) is a testing procedure based on the fact that the superficial major nerves in the body can be electrically stimulated with a bipolar electrode (150 volts, 0.5 msec duration) resulting in depolarization of the nerves and the conduction of an electrical potential. This is recorded on an oscilloscope which shows the latency of the conduction; motor and sensory velocities are established in meters-per-second (Fig. 10).

Reduced motor conduction velocities are usually indicative of a neuropathy. Distal entrapment syndromes, such as the carpal tunnel syndrome, can also be detected. Sensory conduction velocities are important, because in most cases of neuropathy the sensory fibers are affected first, especially in the periphery.

In the upper extremities, the median, ulnar, radial, musculocutaneous, axillary and suprascapular nerves can be tested; in the lower extremities, the peroneal, tibial and femoral nerves are evaluated. At birth the conduction velocities are approximately one-half of the velocities reached at the age of three. The conduction velocities gradually decrease in the decades after the 60th year.

After establishing the motor or sensory conduction velocities of a nerve, a needle electrode (monopolar or concentric) is used

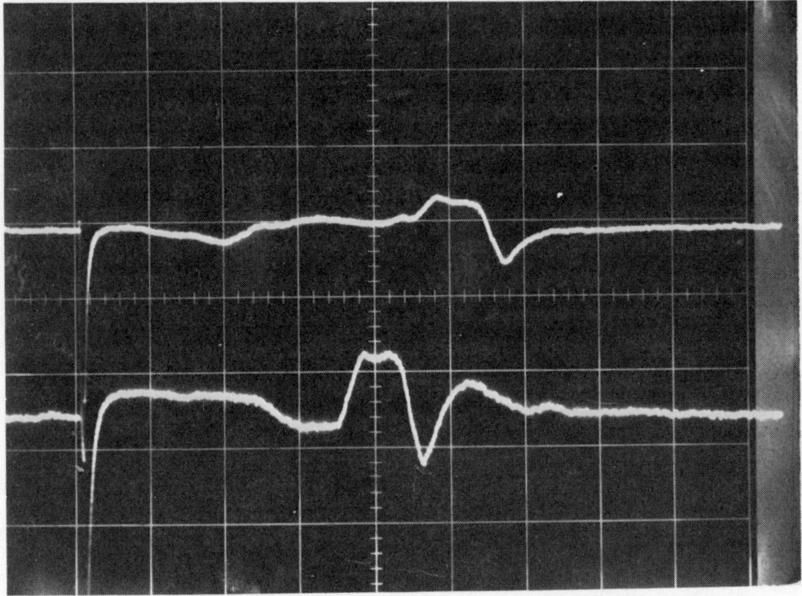

Figure 10.   Measurements of motor conduction velocity in a
45-year-old woman with carpal tunnel syndrome. The action
potential of the opponens pollicis muscle is recorded by disk-
electrode following maximal stimulation of the median nerve
at the elbow (upper tracing) and at the wrist (lower tracing).
Distal motor latency 17.5 m/sec, motor conduction velocity
(elbow-wrist) 50 m/sec. Calibration: each vertical line represents 5 m/sec, each horizontal line 570 μV. (Stimulus artefact
on the left.)

to test the muscle potentials. The relaxed muscle usually gives a
straight line (no potentials) on the oscilloscope without any noise
(through the loud speaker system). Contraction will cause motor-
unit potentials to act. *Polyphasic potentials* with *decreased amplitude* are suggestive of *myogenic* involvement. A *decreased number*
of the motor-unit potentials, with *giant potentials,* is indicative of
a *neurogenic* problem. Fasciculations, fibrillations and positive
waves are suggestive of *denervation.*

In myasthenia gravis, the amplitude of the motor-unit potentials
will gradually decrease after repetitive stimulation (3–6 cycles/sec).

In the Eaton-Lambert syndrome, which occurs with carcinoma of the lung, there will be a facilitating effect before the decrease of the motor-unit potentials occurs.

In myotonia, a repetitive waxing and waning of the motor-unit potentials will occur, usually accompanied by the characteristic sound of a dive bomber or motorcycle.

The test is quite helpful in separating myogenic vs. neurogenic problems, as well as organic from psychogenic involvement of the musculature. A cooperative patient is essential.

Chapter 2

BIRTH DEFECTS AND CONGENITAL MALFORMATIONS

Children may be born with neurologic disorders as well as with disorders involving other organ systems. Often the problems are not accompanied by obvious physical abnormality. For this reason there are various routine tests for examining an infant's neurologic condition. Certain reflexes are usually present at birth and are looked for. Most of these tend to disappear after myelination progresses.

REFLEXES NORMALLY PRESENT AT BIRTH AND INFANCY

- *Moro reflex.* This is the most important of the group. In this reflex the child will flex the arms and legs, as if to embrace the mother, when irritated by loud noises (hand clapping) or vibration (hitting the examining table). The reflex exists up to the age of three or four months and disappears thereafter.

- *Tonic neck reflex.* This also demonstrates the immaturity of the nervous system of the newborn. The infant rests on his back and the head is turned passively to one side. The ipsilateral arm and leg will be extended, the opposite arm and leg flexed. If the baby's head is turned to the opposite side, a reversal of the position of the extremities does occur. The reflex tends to disappear as neural development progresses after a few months.

- *Grasp reflex*. Stimulation of the palm of the hand will result in the child grasping the examiner's finger. This is physiologically present up to the age of three months and weakens thereafter.
- *Babinski phenomenon*. This reflex is physiologically present from birth up to age 16 months and then disappears; it is pathologic in the adult. (See p.14)
- *Spontaneous stepping reflex*. When the child is held in an upright position on the table he will lift one leg (knee flexion) as if stepping. This is usually present from eight weeks to six months of age and disappears later in life.
- *The "parachute" reaction*. Occurs when the child is held one to two feet above the examining table and is then somewhat quickly lowered as though falling. At this time all four limbs will be outstretched as if to cushion the fall.

The foregoing examples represent only a few of the many reflexes which can be studied in the infant, most of which tend to disappear after a few months. The presence or absence of these reflexes as the child grows reflects basic neurologic function, and can indicate both congenital malformations or birth defects. Knowledge of these disorders and their possible sources is important.

CONGENITAL MALFORMATIONS.

These are as follows:

- *Absence of the forebrain* (anencephaly).

- *Absence of the corpus callosum.* This entity is frequently associated with hydrocephalus and mental retardation.
- *Agenesis of one hemisphere with cyst formation.* This usually results in mental retardation and contralateral neurologic signs.
- *Agenesis of the cerebellum* (partial or complete). The individual may learn to function fairly well after several years, thereby overcoming ataxic problems.
- *Hydrocephalus.* The normal circumference of the head at birth is 35 cm. At the age of two the head will have grown to 49 cm. At five a circumference of 52 cm will be reached, indicating a relatively rapid growth of the brain and the encasing bony structures.

A smaller than normal head is called microcephaly; larger than normal is macrocephaly.

Hydrocephalus is the most common cause of macrocephaly and may be congenital or acquired. The *acquired* type is frequently due to infectious diseases (such as meningitis) which obstruct the normal cerebrospinal fluid flow because of adhesions.

Hydrocephalus may also be due to a defect in the absorption of fluid at the arachnoid villi, or to an overproduction of fluid at the choroid plexuses (mainly in the lateral ventricles but also in the third ventricle). Normally the cerebrospinal fluid is exchanged and replaced every 12 to 15 hours.

A *communicating hydrocephalus* is one in which there is a free flow of fluid; the *non-communicating* type is due to obstruction in the passageways, usually at the cerebral aqueduct (Sylvius). Figure 11 is a cast of the ventricular system of the adult human brain viewed from the left side (Sobotta-Figge). More often than not, hydrocephalus is bilateral but can also be unilateral in cases of a defective interventricular foramen (Monro).

In cases of atresia or closure of the median aperture of the fourth ventricle (foramen of Magendie) a Dandy-Walker syndrome results. Atresia of the lateral apertures (foramina of Luschka) may also occur, especially in cases of meningitis.

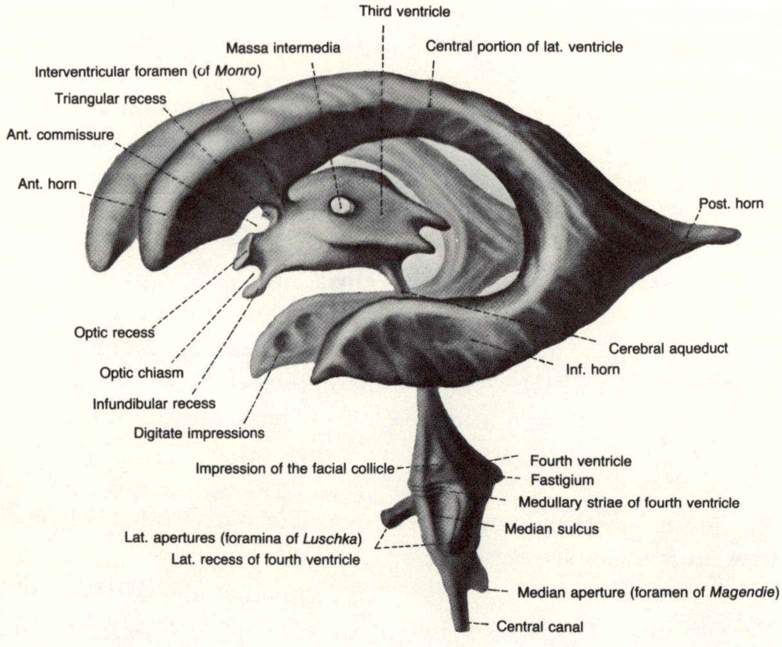

Figure 11.   Cast of the ventricular system of the adult human brain viewed from the left side (from Sobotta-Figge, 1974, Vol 3, Chapter 2, p. 40).

Surgical procedures include draining the spinal fluid into the superior vena cava or into the abdominal cavity in order to reduce the pressure on the brain structures and to avoid cerebral atrophy. To be effective this is done at an early age, preferably before the child is three to four weeks old.

BIRTH DEFECTS

Neurologic defects in neonates may have many sources that are not developmental, but are due to accidents during pregnancy. Prematurely born children, weighing less than five pounds at birth, have a higher incidence of neurologic problems (including epilepsy) than children with normal birth weights (between five and seven pounds). Overdue pregnancies, which may result in a heavier child at birth, have the disadvantage of prolonged labor and a higher incidence of bleeding into the brain structures. Prolonged labor due to a small birth canal may mold the head of the child more severely, thereby causing cerebral abnormalities.

Infantile Cerebral Palsy

These are syndromes occurring before, at, or shortly after birth and for which there are multiple causes. The incidence is approximately 6 per 1000 live births, with a mortality rate of about 10% within the first five years. The main causes are:

- Anoxia of the brain structures
- Hemorrhage into the cerebrum
- Infections affecting the brain or its coverings.

The prenatal and natal occurrences account for approximately 80–90% of all cases, with the remaining 10–20% due to post-natal involvement. In all probability, most cases occur during the prenatal phase of development. Of the various problems that arise the most important cause is *anoxia* of the brain structures, which chiefly involves the gray matter. This can be due to compression of the umbilical cord, or the mother's having prolonged episodes of epileptic seizures, fainting spells or episodes of low blood pressure. Each epileptic spell may cause a temporary arrest of the diaphragm, impair breathing and contribute to lack of oxygen.

Hemorrhages may occur especially in cases of maternal high blood pressure, deficiency of vitamin K (which is especially important in premature births), or in severe accidents to the mother's abdomen. In utero the fetus may be affected by an *infection* of the mother with a neurotropic virus (mumps, measles, chicken pox or influenza). Especially harmful is an infection with rubella (German measles) within the first three months of pregnancy. If the mother has a syphilitic infection the child may be born with congenital lues.

Many *drugs* which are generally used are potentially dangerous to the fetus. In the past the widespread use of Thalidomide resulted in severe and tragic birth defects. Excessive use of *X-rays* and exposure to *atomic radiation* should be avoided during pregnancy. X-ray procedures should be done only when absolutely necessary; all similar diagnostic tests should be postponed until after delivery.

Problems may arise with *incompatibility of the Rh factor. Erythroblastosis fetalis* occurs usually in the second- and third-born child and results in serious complications. One-third of these children die, one-third recover and the remaining third will have serious central nervous system lesions which, in most instances, affect the extrapyramidal tract system and cause marked rigidity and athetosis (slow sinuous movements of the extremities). The treatment in these cases is by blood transfusions.

In the fetus, *toxoplasmosis* causes intracranial calcifications, which can be readily seen on X-rays. *Diabetes mellitus* may result in overweight, with increased size of the fetal head complicating the delivery. Prolonged and severe *liver disease* can cause diminished vitamin K, resulting in bleeding tendencies. *Nutritional difficulties,* possibly related to severe anemia, may result in fetal brain damage, as will repeated episodes of *hypoglycemia* (abnormally low blood glucose).

At birth, *constrictions of the birth canal,* which usually occur with the first born, may cause problems. Violent uterine contractions should be avoided. Drugs such as morphine and barbiturates should be given at delivery only if absolutely necessary. Breech birth may result in severe cerebral anoxia.

The postnatal causes of cerebral palsy that occur within the first week after birth are usually due to infections (birth canal, etc.) to which the child has low resistance.

The localization of the lesions in cerebral palsy syndrome is important. In 60% of the cases the *pyramidal tract* is involved, resulting from bleeding into the parietal lobes and producing spasticity and the so-called "scissors gait." Since mainly the cortex is affected, epilepsy is the frequent result. In 30% of the cases the *extrapyramidal tract system* is involved, with the usual cause being lack of oxygenation of the basal ganglia. Clinically, chorea, athetosis and other hyperkinetic movements may result. In 6% of the cases, basal ganglia system involvement results in rigidity only. The remaining 4% of the infants show cerebellar lesions, which are manifested by marked ataxia.

The primary neurologic impairment of cerebral palsy is frequently accompanied by other problems:

- *Eyes*. Refractive errors and weakness of the eye musculature may occur, as well as clouding of the lens and nystagmus.
- *Epilepsy*. Half of the children have major or minor seizures, due to lesions of the cerebral cortex.
- *Intelligence*. Affected in 50% of the cases, and mental retardation (IQ below 70) occurs.
- *Teeth*. Poor development may be congenital, the problem being complicated, in part, by poor dental hygiene.
- *Speech defects*. These occur in 60% of the children, who will show slurred, disarticulate or spastic speech.
- *Stature*. Children with cerebral palsy tend to be smaller in stature than normal children.
- *Infections*. There is a tendency for the CP child to react more violently to infections (thermal lability); high fever is not uncommon (42–43° C).
- *Emotional problems*. These may arise from frustrations in later life due to the multiplicity of symptoms, or as a result of overprotection by the parents.

Of this group 50% will benefit from rehabilitation procedures, while 25% will not be severely enough affected to need therapy or other methods of rehabilitation. Twenty-five percent will be so severely retarded that in spite of good intentions not much can be achieved through physical or occupational therapy. The rehabilitation goals to strive for are the following:

- Get the child to walk and move about.
- Teach the child to care for himself or herself, so far as eating, dressing, personal hygiene, etc., are concerned.
- Institute communication by speech or writing if possible.
- Dress the child as normally as possible, so that he or she does not appear "different" or socially outcast.

- Adults with CP should have employment within their capabilities, even if only on a part-time basis.
- They should participate in social activities (movies, parties, sports) and, if possible, have some kind of hobby. Occupational therapy is of great importance in the promotion of those skills that are essential to daily living, as well as those that are recreational.

Treatment of the cerebral palsy victim usually involves several specialties: pediatric, orthopedic, psychiatric, and ophthalmologic care. Psychologic studies (for IQ determination) and employment counseling are done. Surgical procedures may have to be resorted to in order to correct contractures at the joints. Motor skills will have to be built up over a period of several years. In some parts of the country, special schools for the mentally retarded and handicapped are operated by the state. The teacher-pupil ratio in these institutions is usually kept low.

Finally, it may be said that with considerable enthusiasm and effort on the part of all concerned great progress on the road to rehabilitation can be made.

Chapter 3

INFECTIOUS DISEASES OF THE BRAIN AND SPINAL CORD

Numerous viral and bacterial diseases attack the central nervous system directly. Infections affecting the brain, due to various agents, are called *encephalitis*. If an infection involves the dura mater a *pachymeningitis* results. More frequently the infection involves the arachnoidea and pia mater, in which case it is called *leptomeningitis* or simply *meningitis*.

The main causes of meningitis are streptococcal, staphylococcal, pneumococcal and meningococcal infections, although in childhood it is frequently caused by *Bacillus coli (B.coli)*. The condition is more apt to occur in children and young adults, and the onset manifests itself with severe headaches, rapidly rising temperatures and pain and stiffness of the neck (nuchal rigidity). Often these symptoms are accompanied by increased intracranial pressure, with vomiting and bradycardia.

In order to establish the diagnosis, a careful spinal tap is done. The fluid may be grayish-yellow and the white blood cell count may be elevated to 300–15,000 cells/cu.mm. *in bacterial meningitis*. The caution in doing the tap is necessary because of possible increased intracranial pressure. Therapy consists mainly of bed rest and antibiotics (penicillin and broad spectrum antibiotics). Fortunately, the mortality rate is low today, although scar formation with adhesions may develop during the acute process and cause symptoms after recovery. Epileptic seizures may result later in life. Most of the bacterial meningitides affect the convexity of the brain; pathologically, a grayish-yellow exudate can be demonstrated.

Tuberculous or fungal infections can cause a meningitis which is likely to involve the base of the brain (basal meningitis). In this condition there is frequent involvement of the cranial nerves (especially VI and VII). The tuberculous type of infection occurs sporadically in this country, but it is still often found in Asian and African countries.

Treatment should be instituted as soon as possible, using either streptomycin, isoniazid or para-aminosalicylic acid. Because of the side effects of streptomycin, which may result in labyrinthine and acoustical changes, these organs should be carefully tested throughout the treatment. It is not always possible to demonstrate the *Mycobacterium tuberculosae* in the spinal fluid, and animal inoculations are frequently needed to verify the tuberculous process.

In cases of bacterial meningitis the organism may not remain in the coverings of the brain but may accumulate within the brain substance and cause *abscesses* of various types, such as cerebral, subdural or extradural. Purulent sinusitis and otitis media are frequent causes for intracerebral brain abscesses in the frontal, or temporal and cerebellar regions. In children with congenital heart abnormalities, where oxygenation of the brain structures is impaired, such infections are much more common than in children free of heart problems.

In any case of meningitis which improves after treatment and then shows sudden deterioration a diagnosis of brain abscess should be considered a possibility. The electroencephalogram will show early changes, (slow waves) although the diagnosis is usually made today by CT-scan. Brain abscesses may also result in patients with lung abscesses, which spread by way of the venous system of the spinal cord to the cranial cavity.

The most serious type of brain infection is *encephalitis* involving the gray matter. Onset is usually associated with lethargy and listlessness in either the child or the adult. The mental capacities deteriorate and seizures may occur, in the beginning with focal characteristics, later generalized.

There are many different types of encephalitis, such as Eastern and Western equine encephalitis (the virus being harbored in the horse), St. Louis encephalitis, herpes simplex encephalitis and inclusion body encephalitis. Since most of these encephalitides are viral in origin, they are more difficult to treat than the bacterial meningitides. The different types of viruses can be isolated in special institutions of viral studies (e.g., Atlanta, Georgia).

Acute anterior poliomyelitis is a viral disease which is now quite rare in the United States; three different types of viruses have been isolated. The symptoms appear in 10 to 12 days after infection and usually in the late summer or fall. Fortunately, the disease is now an uncommon entity. In 1977 twenty paralytic poliomyelitis cases were identified, 14 of them probably vaccine associated. In 1978 only seven paralytic poliomyelitis infections were reported, of which five were probably associated with vaccination. Because of the general immunization of the population this disease is now seen only sporadically throughout the world. At the present time it affects people who have not been immunized and who are in poor health (generally in the older age groups).

The usual onset of the disease is sudden, with cold-like symptoms of fever and muscle aching. After the preparalytic phase the fever may start to rise again. Headaches, pain and tenderness of the musculature develop, and a flaccid muscular paralysis may result. In most instances, the musculature of the lower or upper limbs is affected, but the brain-stem region may be involved, resulting in a high mortality rate (30% in *polioencephalitis*).

In most cases the disease affects the musculature on an asymmetrical basis, mainly the lower extremities, but occasionally the intercostal muscles. The disease process results in a destruction of the anterior horn cells in the spinal cord or, in cases of polioencephalitis, of the cranial nerve nuclei in the brain stem.

The role of the physical therapist is of great importance here to prevent "freezing" of the joints after the acute phase. Passive and active mobilization of the joints and strengthening of the musculature should be done as early as possible. The patient may have to learn to walk again; in the past many patients were confined to a wheelchair or to bed. Rehabilitation of these persons may take months or years.

Other viral infections, such as *rabies,* affect the central nervous system; these usually result from bites by an infected animal (dog, cat, fox, bat, etc.). Spasmodic contractions of the muscles of the mouth, pharynx and larynx are seen in the majority of cases. Spasms of respiratory musculature and convulsive seizures with opisthotonus (arching of the back due to cramping) may also occur. While there is no known treatment of the disease itself, individuals who have been bitten by a suspect animal should undergo immunization therapy immediately.

Chapter 4

CEREBROVASCULAR DISEASES

The leading causes of death in the United States may be summarized as follows:

Age: 15–24 years   1. Accidents (traffic and other injuries)

25–44 years   1. Heart disease
2. Accidents
3. Cancer
4. Cerebrovascular accidents

45–65 years   1. Heart disease
2. Cancer
3. Cerebrovascular accidents

Since the life span is increasing in this country, (1978: men approximately 73 years; women approximately 78 years), these diseases occur more now than before. It is of historical interest that archeological findings in Africa indicate that the human race is about 3.5 million years old, but since the life span was much shorter, CVA was probably relatively unknown then.

Blood supply (Fig. 12). The internal carotid arteries provide two-thirds of the blood supply to the brain, while the vertebro-basilar

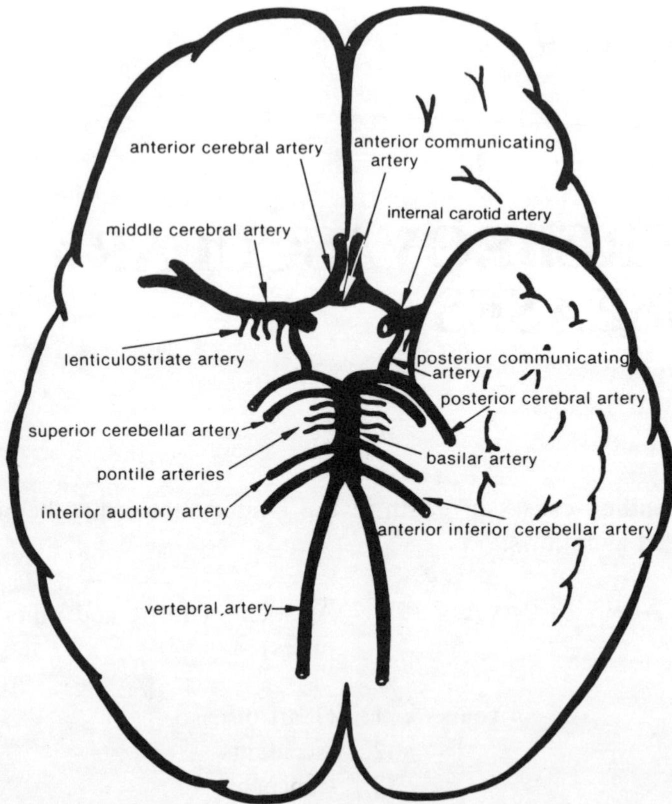

Figure 12.   The arteries of the base of the brain forming the arterial circle.

artery system provides the remainder. Ninety percent of the blood from each cerebral hemisphere is drained by the ipsilateral internal jugular vein; 10% is drained by the contralateral vessel. The blood flow in the cranial vessels can be measured by the use of radioactive material, and the blood flow in the common carotid and vertebral arteries can be determined by Doppler ultrasonic studies.

Arteriosclerosis (pathologic lipid accumulation within the intima) is probably the most common cause of vascular problems. Arteriosclerosis is noticed first and most severe in the main branches of the cerebral vessels, especially in the region of bifurcations and curvatures. For example, the siphon ("S"-shaped curvature) of the internal carotid artery is frequently affected. Basal parts of the larger branches of the middle cerebral arteries are commonly involved, as are arteries going to the basal ganglia. The anterior cerebral artery may be affected where it swings around the corpus callosum. Only in very severe cases are the smaller branches of the convexity involved to the same degree. Diabetes mellitus and hypertension usually enhance arteriosclerosis and cause more pronounced pathologic findings. The following manifestations can be observed:

1. Thrombosis of cerebral arteries with narrowing of the vascular lumen and secondary impairment of blood flow (70–80% of cases).

2. Embolism. Emboli from the heart region may be thrown into the cerebral vessels, where they usually lodge in a vessel at a bifurcation site, abruptly stopping the blood flow (10%). In cases of a patent foramen ovale the embolus could come from the extremities.

3. Hemorrhages frequently occur at "knee bend" sites in an artery, because of constant pounding of the vessel wall by pulsation (especially the lenticulostriate arteries) (15–20%).

4. Vasculitis. Infections with lymphocytic infiltration of the vessel wall can affect cerebral vessels as well as the temporal arteries. Infiltration by lymphocytes and giant cells may occur (giant-cell arteritis).

5. Trauma may result in *extradural* or *subdural hemorrhages* as well as *intracerebral hematomata.* An intracerebral hemorrhage is of sudden onset and is usually accompanied by deep and prolonged unconsciousness.

6. Hypertensive encephalopathy with systolic blood pressure usually above 260mm/Hg and diastolic pressure above 140mm/Hg. With these elevated blood pressure readings the brain starts to swell up (cerebral edema) and this may result in seizures. (The intracranial pressure will, in these cases, exceed the spinal fluid pressure.)

7. Cerebrovascular insufficiency is probably the most frequent consequence of arteriosclerosis to be encountered early and should be treated immediately. Before a thrombosis or complete occlusion of a vessel occurs, the patient may have intermittent episodes of hypoxia. Medical intervention at this stage may prevent a stroke. Cerebrovascular insufficiency can affect all the arteries supplying the brain. A "bruit" (Fr. "brwe") or murmur is heard with the stethoscope over vessels narrowed by more than 50%.

Warning signs for strokes in evolution:

- Episodes of intermittent weakness of one side of the body which become more frequent and of longer duration.

- Episodes of intermittent tingling or numbness of one side of the body, occurring suddenly and becoming more frequent.

- Intermittent blindness (if the arterial narrowing is below the origin of the ophthalmic artery).

- Intermittent speech difficulties (if the dominant hemisphere is involved).

Forty to sixty percent of all strokes are caused by narrowing of the internal carotid artery in the neck region, which is accessible to the vascular surgeon for endarterectomy. Thromboses and hemorrhages occur frequently with generalized arteriosclerosis, hypertension and diabetes mellitus. Arteriosclerosis occurs more frequently at a curved portion of the blood vessel, where turbulence of blood flow is found. A complete arterial occlusion may result in infarction, a wedge-shaped area which becomes necrotic and will be replaced by a cyst containing yellowish fluid, followed by scar-tissue formation (glial cells). In cerebral thrombosis, where the narrowing of the blood vessel occurs gradually, usually a white infarction results. In cases of sudden stoppage of the blood supply (embolus), a red infarction, due to hemorrhage into the damaged area, will occur.

The examination of the stroke patient includes:

1.   History and Occurrence
2.   Appearance of Patient

3. Breathing
4. Consciousness
5. Pulse
6. Spinal Fluid

1. **History and Occurrence.** Thrombosis usually occurs in the older age group (60–80 yrs.), with paralysis occurring overnight, due to stasis of blood flow during sleep in arteries which have already become narrowed. *Cerebroembolism* usually occurs when patients are active and about. *Hemorrhages* classically occur at the height of the day, when the patient is getting somewhat fatigued and is pushing himself.

2 & 3. **Appearance of Patient and Breathing.** In *cerebral thrombosis* the face looks pale and *breathing* is fairly normal, usually. In a sudden event, such as embolism, the face is also pale but breathing is frequently irregular and shallow. In *hemorrhages* the face is usually flushed, the patient is sweating profusely and breathing is usually deep and irregular.

4 & 5. **State of Consciousness and Pulse.** In *cerebral thrombosis* the patient is more apt to be conscious, although he may be drowsy and lethargic. *Pulse* rate is normal or slightly increased. In *embolism* the patient is apt to be sleepy, stuporous and semi-comatose. Pulse rate may be normal or slightly faster than normal. In massive hemorrhages, which have the highest mortality, the patient is usually comatose and unresponsive; the pulse will indicate bradycardia.

6. **Spinal Fluid.** In *cerebral thrombosis* the fluid is usually clear and under normal pressure. With *embolism* the fluid is also usually clear, although a few erythrocytes may be found. The spinal fluid pressure, in most instances, will be normal or minimally elevated. In *cerebral hemorrhage,* depending upon

the site, the fluid is usually grossly bloody and the pressure is markedly elevated. *If blood accumulates in the hemisphere and breaks through into the ventricular system, the prognosis is grave* (because of interference of cerebrospinal fluid circulation).

Narrowing or stenosis of the internal carotid artery. This frequently results in intermittent blindness of the ipsilateral eye and intermittent weakness and numbness of the opposite side of the body. These symptoms usually occur for the first time when the blood vessel is narrowed by approximately 50%. Sometimes a murmur can be heard over the carotid bifurcation. Doppler ultrasonic flow studies and subsequent arteriography may be of help.

Basilar artery insufficiency. Vertigo is the most frequent symptom (lasting a few seconds to a few minutes). Other brain stem signs may include eye muscle weakness and unilateral or bilateral pyramidal tract symptoms. Complete occlusion of the basilar artery is usually not compatible with life, although smaller branches of this vessel may be affected without major problems.

The vertebral arteries may be locally and indirectly affected when a bony spur (in cases of cervical spondylosis) causes pressure on one of the vessels. This can induce a focal arteriosclerosis at the site, leading to vertebral artery stenosis.

A "full-blown stroke" may lead to paralysis of the contralateral arm more than the leg. This occurs in occlusion of the *middle cerebral artery* (80% involvement).

The leg may be more affected than the arm, as in occlusions of the *anterior cerebral artery* (10% involvement).

Ten percent of all hemorrhages occur in the cerebellum without any definite paralysis but with occasional eye movement disorder. A *cerebellar hemorrhage* is surgically accessible and has the best prognosis. The poorest prognosis is with hemorrhages into the lower brain stem, where vital centers (respiration and circulation) are located. A hemorrhage into the pons may result in pinpoint pupils (otherwise seen only in morphinism).

Recently, more arterial thromboses are occurring in young persons, especially females. This increased incidence seems to be related to the prolonged use of birth control pills, although other factors may additionally be responsible. Several syndromes are related to brain stem lesions, usually on a vascular basis:

1. **Weber Syndrome.** A lesion within the area of the nucleus of the oculomotor nerve will cause an ipsilateral eye movement disorder and contralateral affection of the face and extremities.

2. **Benedikt Syndrome.** A lesion within the red nucleus will cause homolateral oculomotor nerve palsy, as well as contralateral hyperkinetic movements in the form of tremor, choreiform movements and athetosis.

3. **Millard-Gubler Syndrome.** A lesion in the posterior part of the pons will cause homolateral facial nerve palsy and a contralateral weakness of the extremities.

4. **Foville Syndrome.** A lesion in the area of the abducens and facial nerves will cause a homolateral paralysis of the muscles concerned and a contralateral weakness of the extremities.

5. **Wallenberg Syndrome.** This is due to a lesion within the posterior inferior cerebellar artery region causing homolateral cerebellar signs in the form of ataxia, a Horner's syndrome (enophthalmos, upper eyelid ptosis, pupillary constriction) on the same side, difficulty in swallowing and a contralateral pain and temperature loss; additional weakness of the musculature occurs in the Babinski-Nageotte syndrome.

Two to three days following the onset of a stroke, passive exercises of the extremities should be done. As soon as the patient is ambulatory, active exercises should be promoted, using rehabilitation facilities. Emphasis should be placed on the avoidance of contractures and on the strengthening of the weakened musculature. This should be continued for several weeks on an outpatient basis following discharge from the hospital.

Chapter 5

HEADACHES (CEPHALGIA)

Headaches are probably the most frequent complaint in clinical neurology. More than 50% of all patients may be bothered by cephalgia. The pain-sensitive structures of the head include, intracranially, the blood vessels (arteries and veins) and the venous sinuses. The brain itself, the dura mater and smaller vessels over the brain surface are insensitive to pain. Extracranial sensitive structures include the periosteum, muscles, skin and cranial nerves carrying afferent pain fibers (V, VII, IX, X, as well as the second and third cervical roots). To diagnose the different types of headaches, a complete and detailed history is mandatory.

It is important to know the location of the ache, the time of onset and the speed of development. Sometimes prodromal signs are present. If the anatomical location can be identified, radiation patterns may be present. In some types of headaches a family history is necessary. The duration of the symptoms is important, as well as the duration of each individual headache. Headache profiles can be established for an individual type (usually in hours) as well as for those occurring over prolonged periods of time (months or years). It is important to know the personality structure of the patient, and whether prior attempts at treatment have been made.

A complete physical and neurologic examination should be done on each patient. Studies may include a complete blood count, glucose level, BUN and liver enzyme studies. X-rays may have to be taken and should include skull films, frequently cervical spine examinations and, in some cases, special views of the sinuses, middle ear and mastoid processes. Refractory errors of the eyes have to be ruled out. Occasionally, further studies such as CT-scan, angiography and spinal fluid examinations may be necessary.

Profile 1—Migraine Headache

This cephalgia is fairly common and most classical, and usually occurs in perfectionistic personalities in managerial positions. Rigid and compulsive mannerisms may be frequently involved. It can occur at any time of the day, but most frequently during the afternoon or evening.

It takes about 20 to 30 minutes to reach its peak and may last for a few hours, sometimes up to two or three days. The headache is described as throbbing or pulsating and usually involves one side of the head at a time. In the next episode the opposite side of the head may be involved; the frontal and temporal regions are preferred.

Sixty percent of patients with migraine have a family history of this condition. There is also a connection with epileptiform disorders; seizures occur more frequently in families with a history of migraine, and migraine occurs more frequently in epileptic families.

In the migraine attack the vessels constrict for a few minutes and then dilate, producing pain.

Ergotamin is the treatment of choice because of its vasoconstrictor capabilities. This drug is contraindicated in pregnancy and renal disease. Usually some caffeine is added (as in Cafergot).

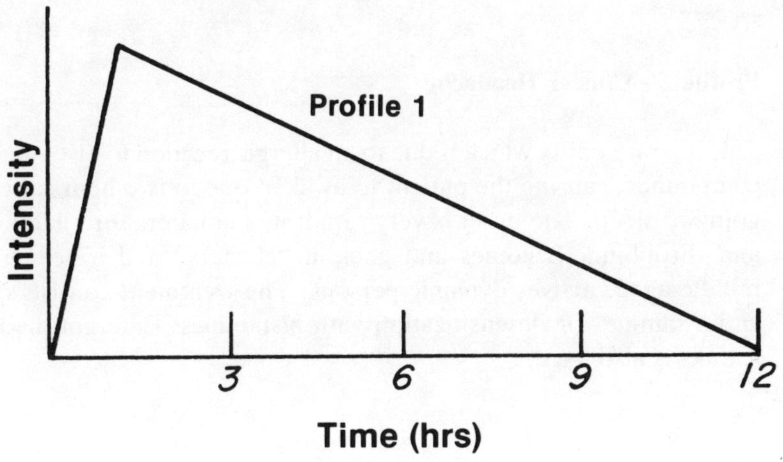

Figure 13.   Migraine headache.

Profile 2—Cluster Headache

This is a rare entity which is due to an allergic reaction to histamine compounds, causing the patient to awaken one to two hours after going to sleep. The onset is very rapid: it is unilateral or bilateral and throbbing. It comes and goes in "clusters" and is seen in middle-aged, active, dynamic persons. The treatment consists of antihistamines or desensitization with histamines; Cafergot medication is also used.

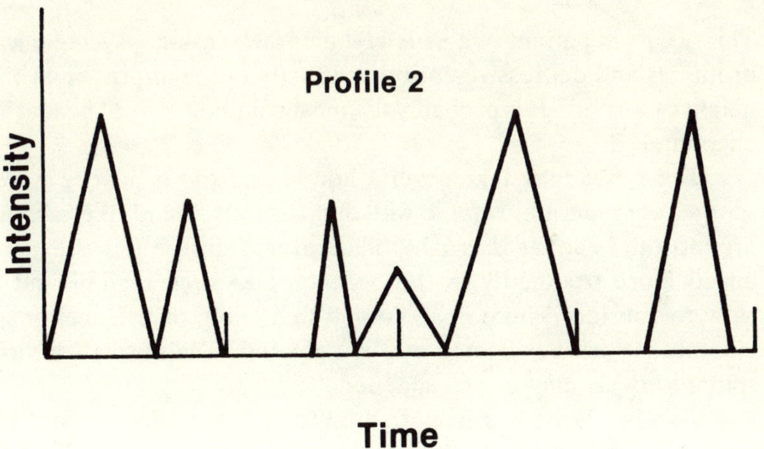

Figure 13.   Cluster headache.

Profile 3—Tension Headache

This occurs in patients with anxiety, nervous tension, psychological problems and depressive episodes, usually in the afternoon at the height of activity. It is probably the most common type of headache encountered.

The onset may take several hours, and the headache is described as moderately severe with deep, steady "band-like" aching around the head. It is usually bilateral and diffuse but is experienced more frequently in the occipital and neck regions and is slow to subside. There is additional tightening of the neck musculature, which can sometimes be palpated. The normal cervical spinal lordosis may be straightened.

This headache is usually treated for a few weeks by sedatives or minor tranquilizers such as Valium or Librium; analgesics may also be used. Psychiatric treatment may sometimes be necessary, especially if there are major psychological problems.

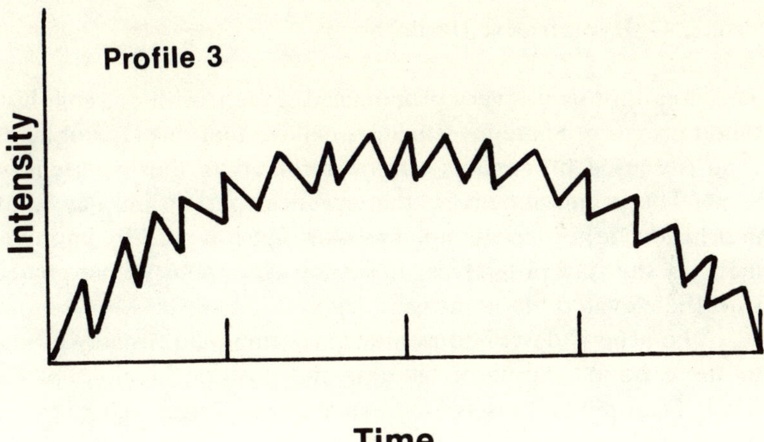

Figure 13.   Tension headache.

Profile 4—Hypertensive Headache

This condition is not very pronounced, except with extreme high blood pressure. Some investigators believe that this type of headache is caused by nervous tension rather than the hypertension itself. The common belief is that severe hypertension may result in a headache, especially upon awakening, followed by improvement as the day progresses; it is, however, poorly coordinated with the elevated blood pressure level.

The ache is described as a deep, boring pain, usually of one to three hours' duration, favoring the posterior regions of the head. Treatment consists of antihypertensive drugs, analgesics and sedatives.

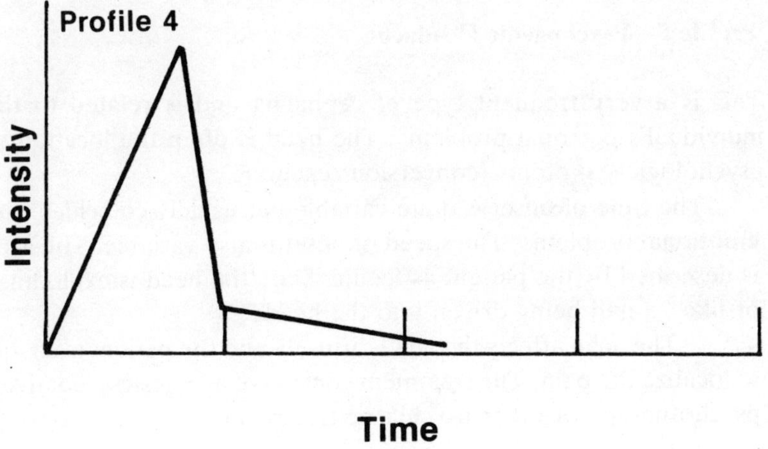

Figure 13.   Hypertensive headache.

Profile 5—Psychogenic Headache

This is a very frequent type of cephalgia and is related to the individual's personal problems. The head is often the location of psychologic symptoms (conversion reaction).

The time of onset is quite variable but usually coincides with emotional problems. The speed of onset is also variable. The ache is described by the patient as feeling like "the head is exploding" or like "a nail being driven into the head."

The ache affects the head diffusely and the patient is unable to localize the pain. The treatment consists of analgesics, sedatives, psychotherapy or other psychiatric treatment.

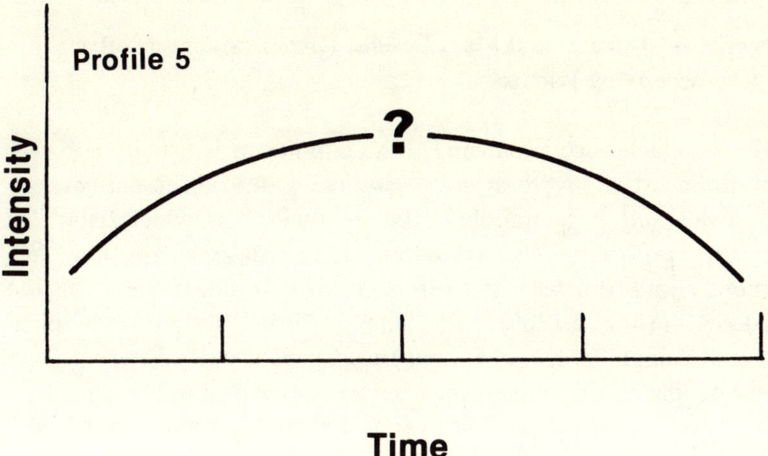

Figure 13.   Psychogenic headache.

Profile 6—Intracranial Mass Lesions (Brain tumors or other space-occupying lesions)

The headache accompanying these conditions is usually not very pronounced or severe in the beginning. Later on the patient may be awakened in the middle of the night with pain which lasts from one to two hours. The frontal and temporal areas are more frequently involved with the cephalgia usually being found on the side of the lesion (80%). The aching can be brought on by positional changes of the head and the pain is usually different from any headache the patient may have experienced in the past. The treatment is by surgical intervention (craniotomy) after the condition has been thoroughly investigated. (See chapter on tumors.)

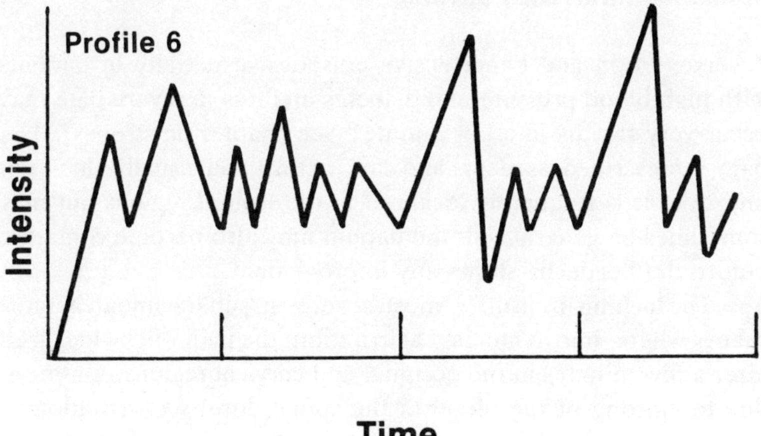

Figure 13.   Headache of space-occupying lesions.

Profile 7—Intracranial Bleeding

After exertion and hypertensive episodes, especially in patients with high blood pressure and diabetes mellitus, a severe pain may occur very rapidly in a few minutes (see chapter on strokes). The pain is described as deep and lancinating and usually does not improve. It is frequently localized in the frontal regions but may sometimes be generalized; the patient may also become comatose before the headache shows any improvement.

The aching is usually most severe in subarachnoid hemorrhages where, due to meningeal irritation, the pain will be localized after a few minutes in the occipital and cervical regions. Later on, due to clotting of the blood in the spinal dural sac, irritation of the lumbar roots may occur with pain radiating into the legs. The treatment is usually initially conservative but may require subsequent surgical intervention.

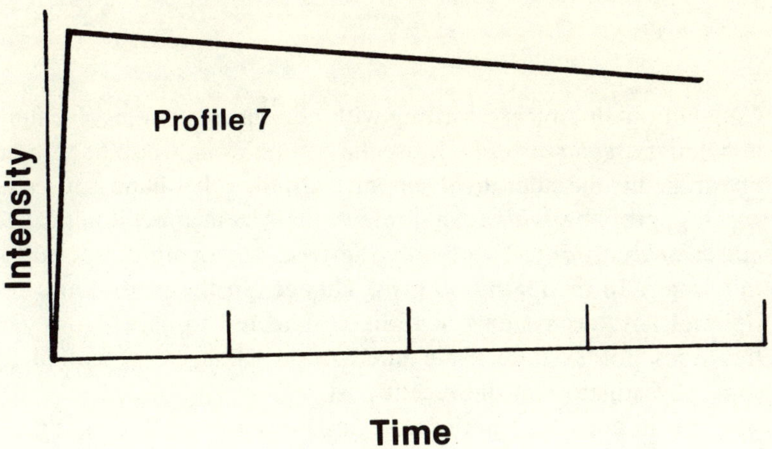

Figure 13.   Headache of intracranial bleeding.

Chapter 6

MUSCULAR DISEASES

Atrophies and Dystrophies

Conventionally, muscle wasting with nervous system involvement is called *muscular atrophy*. Muscular atrophies may also be termed "neurogenic muscular involvement." On the other hand, muscular wasting, probably *without* major nervous system affection, is called *muscular dystrophy*. Frequently the term "myopathy" is used for this latter. In myopathy no gross changes in the central and peripheral nervous systems have been detected to date. However, this does not exclude some microscopic changes, described by some investigators in the recent past.

It is important to notice that these diseases tend to be diffuse and symmetrical in their spread, but at the onset, one side may be affected more than the other; there is no sensory loss. Hereditary factors are often present and infections and trauma are unlikely causes. While enzyme deficiency may be the causative factor in several of these conditions, the most commonly accepted theory is that they are disorders of metabolism resulting in faulty oxygenation and nutrition of muscle tissue. Other neurophysiologic and biochemical processes may be involved. In some of these entities we still do not understand the basic biochemical processes underlying the abnormal states, and therefore we use descriptive terms to correlate the clinical findings with the anatomical structure in regard to pathological lesions. When these diseases are more fully understood they probably will be reclassified according to etiology.

DIFFERENTIAL DIAGNOSIS AND LOCALIZATION

(Note: For this and the discussion which follows refer to Figure 14). The differentiation between upper and lower motor neuron diseases is quite important and should be fully understood. The following entities will be considered:

1. Progressive Spastic Bulbar Paralysis (Duchenne), also frequently called pseudobulbar palsy in clinical terms.
2. Progressive Spastic Spinal Paralysis.
3. Amyotrophic Lateral Sclerosis (ALS).
4. Progressive Bulbar Palsy.
5. Progressive Spinal Muscular Atrophy (Werdnig-Hoffmann's disease).
6. Amyotonia Congenita (Oppenheim's disease).
7. Progressive Neuropathic (Peroneal) Muscular Atrophy (Charcot-Marie-Tooth disease).
8. Progressive Hypertrophic Interstitial Neuropathy (Dejerine-Sottas disease).
9. Myasthenia Gravis and Myasthenic Syndrome (Eaton-Lambert).
10. Muscular Dystrophy of the Atrophic Type (Leyden) and Pseudohypertrophic Type (Duchenne).
11. Myotonia Congenita (Thomsen's disease).
12. Dystrophia Myotonica (Steinert's disease).
13. Familial Periodic Paralysis (due to potassium deficiency).
14. Myositis.

A. UPPER MOTION NEURON DISEASES

1. Progressive Spastic Bulbar Paralysis (Duchenne)

In this entity there is interruption of the intracerebral corticobulbar and corticospinal tracts bilaterally. This can occur in cases of bilateral cerebral vascular accidents, in bilateral demyelinating processes (as in multiple sclerosis) and in amyotrophic lateral sclerosis.

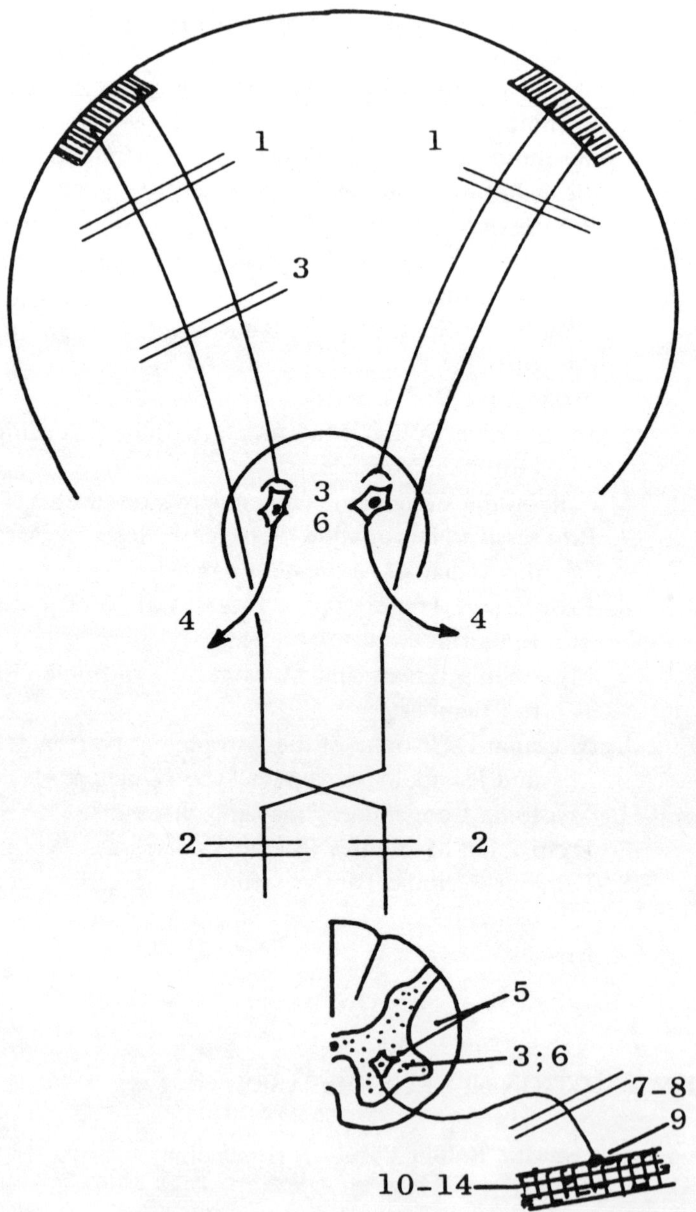

Figure 14.   Neurologic areas involved in muscular atrophies and dystrophies. Numbers refer to entities discussed in text.

The patients exhibit difficulty in speaking, swallowing and spasticity of the extremities; memory is involved to some degree. There is lack of emotional control, with excessive laughter or crying. The prognosis is guarded; survival is usually one to two years, with death commonly occurring from aspiration. Conservative measures such as tube feeding and nursing care are required.

2. Progressive Spastic Spinal Paralysis

This is a condition in which the pyramidal tract fibers in the spinal cord are affected, usually bilaterally. It occurs in amyotrophic lateral sclerosis, multiple sclerosis or vitamin B_{12} deficiency. The process progresses slowly and may last for many years and may occur at the cervical, thoracic or lumbar spinal levels. If the cervical cord is involved, the upper and lower extremities may become spastic; if the thoracic level is involved, the upper extremities may be spared. There is no specific treatment available and nursing care should be directed toward the avoidance of decubitus and other infections.

B. COMBINED UPPER AND LOWER MOTOR NEURON DISEASES

3. Amyotrophic Lateral Sclerosis (ALS)

This is a condition, first described by Charcot, which involves both the upper and lower motor neurons; males are affected slightly more than females. The age of onset is between 40–60 years and wasting of the intrinsic muscles of the hand usually occurs first, followed by spasticity of the musculature of the extremities. Muscle fasciculations can be observed and in the EMG fibrillations and positive waves (denervation potentials) are present; there is a very slight reduction in motor conduction velocities beyond the reduction seen in advancing age.

The survival time depends upon the location of the lesion. If the brain stem is involved, the survival time is six months to two years; if the spinal cord is primarily affected, the survival time may be three to five years. This is a disease of unknown etiology with no specific treatment; proper nursing care and prevention of infection are the primary goals. (See page 106.)

C. LOWER MOTOR NEURON DISEASES

4. Progressive Bulbar Palsy

This is a neurologic entity of extremely poor prognosis, the survival time being around four to six months. The usual cause of death is aspiration pneumonia. The tongue is atrophic (as seen on the floor of the mouth) and shows contractions without purpose (fasciculations).

5. Progressive Spinal Muscular Atrophy (Werdnig-Hoffmann's Disease)

This condition, which tends to be symmetrical, is seen in infants, usually normal at birth, beginning in the sixth to eighth month of life. The child may never learn to walk at all and the longest survival time reported is to the age of six years. No specific treatment is available at this time.

6. Amyotonia Congenita (Oppenheim's Disease)

The lesion here is usually at the anterior horn cell level. This entity is more benign than the previous one, there being a 75% survival rate. The onset is in infancy at the age of six to eight months. After two years of slowly progressing symptoms, there is usually no further progression; it is possible that a slight improvement may occur. No specific treatment is available but physical therapy is recommended to overcome the muscular weakness.

7. Progressive Neuropathic (Peroneal) Muscular Atrophy (Charcot-Marie-Tooth Disease).

In this disease the peripheral nerves are mainly involved (segmental demyelination). There is a strong hereditary factor (dominant inheritance) present, with the onset usually occurring at the age of fifteen to twenty years. Motor and sensory fibers of peripheral nerves are affected and the conduction velocity is markedly reduced, to approximately 20m/sec. Bilateral foot drop and "stork-like walk" (also called "steppage gait") are characteristic.

The anterior horn cells and the posterior columns are involved as well. The peroneal musculature is primarily affected but later on the disease spreads to affect the intrinsic muscles of the feet and hands. Physical therapy and orthopedic applications will be required to support the dropped foot. The prognosis is relatively good and the disease progresses very slowly.

8. Progressive Hypertrophic Interstitial Neuropathy (Dejerine-Sottas Disease)

This is another condition in which a hereditary factor is involved. Nodular thickening of the endoneurium is present and numbness and tingling of the hands and feet occur, together with muscular weakness and wasting. The hypertrophic nerves (peroneal and ulnar which are situated superficially) can be palpated but are not tender. The myelin sheath may be partially destroyed and the axon cylinders are affected; reflexes are usually diminished or absent. The disease progresses very slowly and the prognosis is relatively good. Usually a normal life-span can be expected. Treatment is directed toward combating contractures.

D. NEUROMUSCULAR JUNCTION INVOLVEMENT

9. Myasthenia Gravis and Myasthenic Syndrome (Eaton-Lambert)

The condition is one of an acetylcholine deficiency at the neuromuscular junction due to an increase in the enzyme acetylcholine esterase (cholinesterase), resulting in an impairment of synaptic transmission. The onset is usually in the third decade, with 60% of the cases occurring between the ages of 20 to 24. Occurrences in the newborn and in the sixth decade have been reported. Both sexes are equally vulnerable and in women 50% of the patients have an enlarged thymus gland; therefore, an autoimmune process may be superimposed.

Clinically, weakness of the eye muscles is apparent quite early and ptosis of the eyelids may occur. Difficulties in swallowing, speaking and breathing are frequently noted and the peripheral muscles may be involved; there is usually no atrophy, however. The symptoms tend not to be as pronounced in the morning as in the evening, after the musculature has been used during the day. Neostigmine is the specific drug for treatment; Mestinon and cortisone are also used.

In myasthenia gravis the EMG-testing reveals a gradual reduction in the amplitude of the motor-unit potentials when repetitive stimulation (3–6 cycles/sec) is used. In the *Myasthenic Syndrome* there is a facilitating effect before the decrease of the motor-unit potentials occurs.

If a thymoma is present surgical intervention may become necessary. The tensilon test is used to see whether the impaired muscles respond; recurring muscle strength is quickly achieved but of short duration (minutes). In myasthenia gravis some muscular wasting may be found in the end stages of the disease.

The myasthenic syndrome occurs with oat-cell carcinoma of the lung, as well as with other types of carcinomas, and mainly affects the proximal musculature of the extremities. Neostigmine is of *no* value in this condition, although guanidine may be used with some benefit.

E. SKELETAL (STRIATED) MUSCLE INVOLVEMENT

10. Muscular Dystrophy of the Atrophic Type (Leyden) and Pseudohypertrophic Type (Duchenne)

The muscular dystrophies have an early onset, they are progressive and they are usually hereditary. Females are frequently slightly more involved than males, and death is usually due to respiratory muscular weakness (intercostal and diaphragmatic).

Muscular dystrophies usually affect the proximal muscles more than the distal, except in the Gower's type, where the distal muscles of the arms and legs are primarily involved. In muscular dystrophy the patient usually has a marked lumbar lordosis with "waddling gait". He has difficulty getting up from the floor and has to "climb up on his own legs." Also to be seen are a myopathic face with drooping of the eyelids and difficulty in closing the lips firmly. Usually, creatine phosphokinase in the blood is elevated and reflexes are diminished or absent.

In the *Pseudohypertrophic Type* of the disease, which affects mainly boys, the disease usually starts before the age of five years. The patient has the waddling type of gait (duck-like) and, more often than not, the gastrocnemius and soleus muscles are hypertrophic due to fat accumulation.

There is also a muscular dystrophy affecting just the eye muscles (ocular myopathy), and in longstanding dystrophies the myocardium may be affected. The prognosis, in most cases, is fair, although the life span may be shortened by ten to twenty years.

In the *Atrophic Type* marked muscle wasting is noted, sometimes affecting mainly the shoulder and pelvic girdle musculature or that of the limbs.

Many sub-types of muscular dystrophy have been identified. The electromyogram reveals the *amplitude* of the motor-unit potentials to be *markedly diminished* in myopathy, while the *number* of the motor-unit potentials *remains unchanged.* In contrast, in neurogenic disease the amplitude may even be increased (giant potentials), and the number may be moderately decreased. Since no specific treatment is available for the muscular dystrophies, physical and occupational therapy goals should be directed toward strengthening and preserving the affected musculature.

11. Myotonia Congenita (Thomsen's Disease)

This is an entity which affects the relaxation of the musculature. It is hereditary (autosomal dominant) and a relatively rare condition in which the peripheral muscles in the arms and legs are chiefly affected. Pathophysiologically it is thought to reflect impairment of the muscle membrane. The patient develops an inability to relax as well as an inability to use the muscles quickly. Reflexes are normal and no muscle wasting is observed; on the contrary, the muscles are well developed. Mild mental abnormalities can also be found. Paramyotonia occurs in normal individuals when the temperature is low, but after a warm-up period the muscles can be used effectively.

12. Dystrophia Myotonica (Steinert's Disease)

This is a rare, inherited condition (mainly autosomal dominant) in which there is also an increase in muscle tone. The basic metabolic rate is decreased and there is an increased incidence of cataracts and testicular atrophy. Profound frontal baldness is frequently seen. The life span is decreased by about twenty years, with death usually due to infections.

Most frequently involved are the sternocleidomastoid and other muscles of the neck. Early involvement of the face musculature is common. Later on, atrophy of the peripheral muscles, with a myotonic component, occurs. The myotonic component usually precedes the atrophic process. Most of the patients are found to have a relatively low level of intelligence. Rehabilitation therapy and quinine hydrochloride treatment have been used.

13. Familial Periodic Paralysis

This condition is due to a potassium deficiency and can be treated by administration of potassium chloride. It is a rare condition and death may occur from respiratory paralysis. Usually the patient experiences extreme muscle weakness for hours. After administration of potassium chloride orally the strength of the muscles quickly returns. Potassium deficiencies due to the use of diuretics can also produce a similar syndrome.

14. Myositis

This is a lymphocytic infiltration of the muscle and sometimes also of the skin (dermato-myositis). The disease frequently occurs in middle life and may be associated with carcinoma, especially of the pancreas. The prognosis is guarded (because of the frequent presence of a carcinoma) and only 50% of the cases recover.

In the acute stage the patient may need absolute bed rest in a relatively warm room, and excellent care of the skin should be given to avoid decubitus; aspirin may also be needed. In the acute stage some temperature elevations occur, which subside later. The muscles are painful on palpation and weakness develops, the proximal muscles being more involved than the distal.

During the period of painful muscular swelling there is local tenderness and possibly subcutaneous edema with skin rashes. In the biopsy specimen the muscles are grossly pale and swollen and reveal cellular infiltrates; later on, fiber replacement occurs. Treatment by penicillin, cortisone and adrenocorticotropic hormone (ACTH) is recommended. In the subacute stage massage and exercises may be used. After treatment by long-term rehabilitation procedures the patient may improve considerably.

Chapter 7

EXTRAPYRAMIDAL TRACT DISEASES

Extrapyramidal system anatomy is outlined in Figure 15. All of the areas in the diagram are interconnected in the brain stem. Fibers from the red nucleus continue down into the spinal cord as the rubrospinal tract, probably to the anterior horn cells. Recent neurochemical studies have shown that dopamine is a substance produced by, and accumulated in, the substantia nigra. The chemical substance is then transferred to other structures in the extrapyramidal system (i.e., lentiform and caudate nuclei). Pathologic changes of the substantia nigra result in a depleted, or diminished, reservoir of dopamine. This in turn will cause major effects on the entire extrapyramidal system.

The globus pallidus is regarded as a reservoir of movement impulses. Lesions here therefore result in diminished movement. Slower and less detailed motions (akinesis or hypokinesis) occur. The putamen and caudate nucleus, on the other hand, have an inhibiting and diminishing effect on the muscle tone. An anatomical lesion therefore results in an increase in body movement (hyperkinesis). All of the involuntary movements, such as tremor, chorea, athetosis and ballismus (violent movements of the extremities), disappear in sleep and can be observed only in the waking state. All of the following are associated with extrapyramidal tract involvement.

1. Parkinson's Disease (Paralysis Agitans)

The causes of this syndrome are manifold.

- Idiopathic (probably one of the most frequent).
- Encephalitic (usually observed after von Economo's encephalitis).
- Carbon monoxide poisoning (intoxication from operating internal combustion engines, gas stoves, etc. in unventilated areas).
- Manganese poisoning (industrial).
- Arteriosclerosis (usually in elderly patients).
- Tranquilizing drugs, especially the major tranquilizers such as Compazine, Stelazine and Haldol (the most frequent cause of Parkinsonism in institutions).

The pathologic lesions in this disease are mainly in the substantia nigra and the globus pallidus, causing a deficiency of dopamine, as noted before. The finer movements of the hands are usually involved first. The patient notices difficulties in buttoning or unbuttoning shirts, or in lacing and unlacing shoes, and he walks in a short-stepped gait with difficulty in maintaining his balance.

Other hallmarks of the disease include the following:
- "Pill-rolling tremor" of the fingers (frequency of 5–6 cycles/sec).
- Overestimation of unknown weight placed in patient's hand (in cerebellar disease weight is underestimated).
- Tendency of the handwriting to get smaller and show evidence of tremor. (Tremor on movement is seen in cerebellar disease but with *larger* handwriting.)
- Mask-like face and slower response of facial expression.

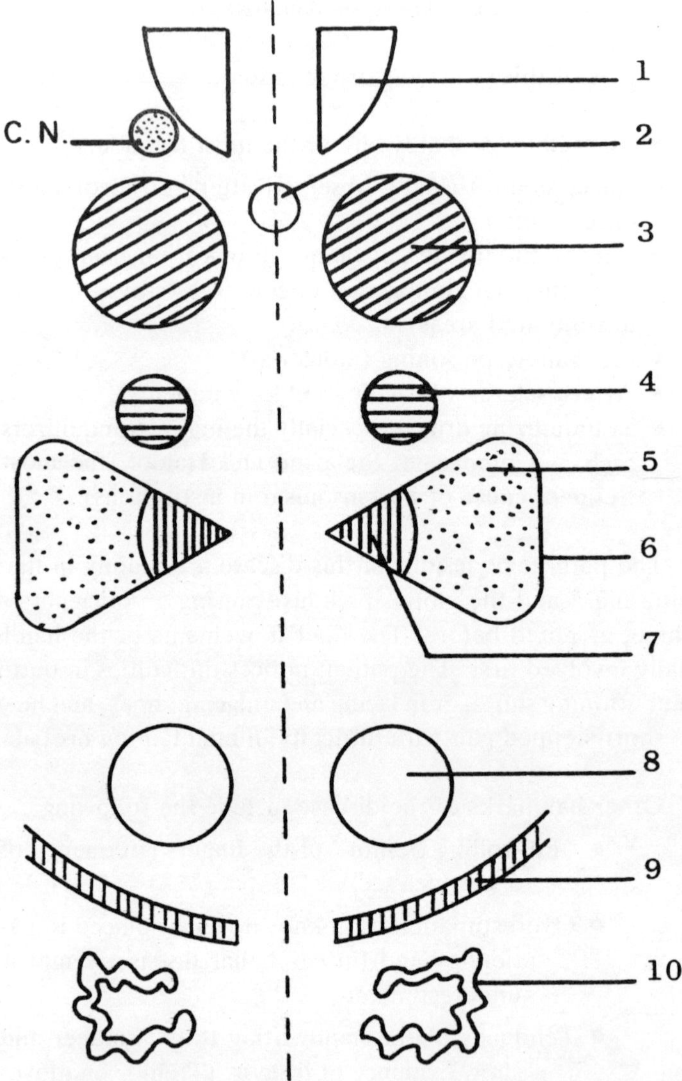

Figure 15.   Diagram of extrapyramidal system anatomy. 1. Lateral ventricle; 2. Third ventricle; 3. Thalamus; 4. Subthalamic nucleus; 5. Putamen; 6. Lentiform nucleus; 7. Globus pallidus; 8. Red nucleus; 9. Substantia nigra (dopamine reservoir); 10. Olive; C.N. Head of caudate nucleus.

- "Cogwheel rigidity" can be observed in more advanced cases. Movements are slow and of limited range because the antagonists are not completely relaxed. (Increased range of movements with decreased tone is seen in cerebellar disease.)

- Patient may suffer from day-night disturbances. He is extremely tired during the day and rather restless during the night.

- Difficulty in keeping position if pushed forward, backward or to the side (antero-posterior and lateral pulsion).

- Diminished mental reactions. In early Parkinsonism this is often *misdiagnosed* as depression.

- Development of an oculogyric crisis. This can occur in post-encephalitic Parkinsonism as well as in cases caused by tranquilizing drugs. Here the patient notices painful movements of the eyes to one side or up and down, lasting a few minutes. The patient may also not be able to converge his eyes.

- Drooling from the mouth. This is seen especially in post-encephalitic and drug-induced cases. All the major tranquilizers such as Compazine, Stelazine, Thorazine and Haldol may cause these drug-related symptoms.

The treatment of Parkinsonism consists of L-dopa, 300–500 mg. per day. L-dopa is converted to dopamine in the brain. Dopamine is not effective, hence only the precursor, L-dopa, can be used. This treatment is somewhat less helpful in severe cases and after the age of 50–60 years. Side effects, such as nausea and vomiting, may occur. Usually the patients improve rather rapidly and have to be guarded against sudden overtaxing of the heart after improvement with L-dopa. The medication has to be taken for life, since the treatment is only a substitution for dopamine deficiency. The effectiveness of the therapy gradually decreases.

A combination of carbidopa and levodopa (Sinemet) is now frequently used; the side effects will be less pronounced because of the lower amounts of L-dopa. Most patients can be maintained on three to six tablets of Sinemet (125–250 mg/day), given in divided doses. It has been found that amantadine-HCl (Symmetrel), which is not related to levodopa or anticholinergic anti-Parkinsonism drugs, has benefits. The usual dose of Symmetrel is 100 mg. twice a day. Occasionally patients may benefit from an increase up to 400 mg. daily. Other drugs can be used in combination with Symmetrel; Artane (2 and 5 mg.) two to three times daily has been used in the past, and occasionally the patient improves after the use of the antihistaminic Benadryl (Artane and Benadryl are not as potent as the drugs described above). At times, stereotactical operations using coagulation or freezing, which interrupt the extrapyramidal pathways, are performed unilaterally and may be of help (thalamotomy). Physical and occupational therapy play a major role in the management of Parkinsonism. The patient may benefit by playing with a ball, building blocks or squeezing a sponge. Finer movements have to be relearned. The patient has to be retrained in walking, ascending stairs and in avoiding abrupt turning movements. He should also be taught to enlarge his limited range of movement.

2. Tics

These are sudden, purposeless movements localized to a particular muscle group. The face, neck or arms are the most frequent sites. Tics are commonly caused by psychological factors, although 10% can be related to sequelae of encephalitis or severe head injuries. Symptoms may last a lifetime, usually reflect psychogenesis and can readily be noticed by others if they affect the face. Tics disappear during sleep. Treatment is very difficult; minor tranquilizers may occasionally be of help.

3. Spasmodic Torticollis (Torticollis Spasticus)

The majority of cases are probably due to psychogenic problems. The head will jerk to one side and, subsequently, the sternocleidomastoid muscle tends to hypertrophy on the side opposite to which the head is turned; this occurs after prolonged involvement. Ten percent of the cases may be due to encephalitis with basal ganglia involvement in the past. No major pathologic lesions have been demonstrated in many cases. The wearing of a neck collar may be of help, and minor tranquilizers can be used. Psychotherapy is usually in order and may be of major benefit. It is interesting to note that sometimes the touching of the face by a finger only will prevent the grotesque-looking, jerky movements of the head.

4. Huntington's Chorea

This is a condition marked by facial grimacing, explosive speech, memory loss and major involuntary movements of choreiform or athetoid type. Choreatic movements are sudden, lightning-like contractions of skeletal muscles; athetosis consists of slow and sinuous movements of the extremities, especially marked in the forearm. In this disease the caudate nucleus is affected and, because of the atrophy, the lateral ventricles become enlarged, especially in the lower portions. This can be demonstrated by CT-scan or pneumoencephalography. The electroencephalogram (EEG) will reveal a low-amplitude waking and sleep record. The disease is autosomal-dominantly inherited but the onset is usually at the age of 30–50 years and the patient will gradually become demented. (Cases of juvenile onset are known). *This disease has the highest suicidal rate of all neurological entities* because of the patient's probable foreknowledge of his physical and, especially, mental deterioration.

Huntington's chorea may have originated in England and southern Denmark, and many immigrants on Long Island (NY) and in Michigan are affected. Since the disease rarely manifests itself before the age of 40 years, and because of its genetic nature, it poses a major problem with individuals whose children have already come along. Hence, genetic counseling may be of help. Eventually the patient will have difficulty walking, feeding and dressing himself and usually ends up as a demented patient in an institution. No specific treatment is available; Haldol can be given.

5. Sydenham's Chorea

This is a non-inherited condition and usually follows streptococcal throat infections, scarlatina or rheumatic fever. It occurs mainly in young people, and the symptoms clear up in a relatively short time (six months). The patient may have to be kept on penicillin for a long time after the onset to avoid possible heart damage due to the streptococcal infection (sometimes for as long as 2–10 years).

6. Chorea Gravidarum

This is a benign condition which usually disappears after pregnancy is terminated. Some researchers believe that it is actually Sydenham's chorea occurring during pregnancy. Some of these choreatic patients are, at first, thought to be overly nervous, and for this reason the disease is frequently missed at the beginning.

7. Ballismus

A syndrome manifested by extraordinary, wide-ranged movements of the arms and legs. It often affects only one side of the body (hemiballismus). The cause is usually arteriosclerotic-thrombotic lesions in the subthalamic nucleus (Luysii). If the condition is bilateral, it poses a threat to survival because of the great expenditure of energy in continuous muscular activity during the day. The metabolic rate is increased considerably. The patient is unable to walk, feed or dress himself. The condition is usually seen in older persons; it is helped to some degree by sedatives and tranquilizers.

8. Hepato-Cerebral Degeneration   (Hepatolenticular degeneration or Wilson's Disease)

In this entity the liver is involved, with subsequent cirrhosis; both the liver and the spleen are enlarged. The onset is usually between 10 and 20 years of age. The patient exhibits a "wing-beating" tremor, a violent arm-flapping movement as seen in birds. The disease is aggravated by nervous tension and anxiety, as are all extrapyramidal tract diseases. The probable cause is a defect in copper metabolism. An increased deposition of copper will be found in the basal ganglia, liver, spleen, urine and stool.

Especially characteristic of the condition is the Kayser-Fleischer ring, which represents a copper accumulation in Descemet's membrane of the cornea. The brownish-gray ring can be seen with the naked eye or by split-lamp examination. The cause of copper accumulation may be the diminished ceruloplasmin of the blood, although other mechanisms may also be involved. The disease is recessively inherited on an autosomal basis and can be treated with Penicillamine, which removes the copper deposition. The life expectancy is usually 10 to 15 years less than normal, in spite of treatment. Before Penicillamine was used, British anti-lewisite (BAL) was the drug of choice but the results were less effective; these two drugs are known as chelating agents.

Chapter 8

METABOLIC AND TOXIC DISORDERS

A. METABOLIC DISORDERS

1. Diabetes Mellitus. The increased sugar content of the blood (hyperglycemia) may cause a non-painful neuropathy, especially of the sensory fibers of the peripheral nerves in arms and legs. The first symptom is usually tingling and numbness of the distal parts of the lower extremities. The distal parts of the upper extremities may become involved as well. (See page 88.)

It is not unusual to find the eye musculature, especially that supplied by the oculomotor nerve (Cr.N.III), also involved. The trochlear and abducens nerves (IV and VI) are less frequently affected. Primarily the vasa nervorum are involved, with the nerves being affected secondarily. An axonal degeneration can be demonstrated by microscopic examination.

Usually the patients have had diabetes mellitus for a considerable time, but there is no definite correlation between the time of onset, the duration and the severity of diabetes with peripheral nerve involvement.

2. Porphyria. This is an inherited inborn error of metabolism in which the patient excretes uroporphyrin in the urine and feces. The urine has a port-wine-red color and hematuria has to be ruled out. This is a painful neuropathy and may be accompanied by seizures and psychosis with visual hallucinations. Abdominal pains are the hallmark of this disease and therefore it is frequently misdiagnosed as a gastrointestinal problem, resulting in abdominal surgery. No specific treatment is available at this time.

3. Phenylketonuria (PKU). This condition is the first of the inborn errors causing dementia to be identified, and it may cause a preventable mental retardation. All the newborn in this country are tested for this in the first three or four days of life (Guthrie test). Diagnosing the disease early and treating it during the first few weeks of life is of the utmost importance in order to prevent mental retardation. In this disease phenylalanine cannot be metabolized, because of the lack of phenylalanine hydroxylase. The treatment, in general, consists of a low ketone diet.

4. Maple sugar urine disease. This is a relatively rare inborn error of amino acid metabolism involving a deficiency of the amino acids leucine, isoleucine and valine. The patient may show mental retardation as well as convulsions, and death usually ensues in a short period of time.

5. Galactosemia. In this inborn error of metabolism the patient cannot metabolize the carbohydrate galactose. The condition leads to severe mental retardation, epileptic seizures and death if untreated. Even with treatment, the patient will remain slightly galactosemic throughout life. High amounts of galactose in the blood and urine can be demonstrated. The treatment consists of soybean preparations taken in a formula. The patient's condition can be improved slightly.

6. Tay-Sachs Disease (cerebro-macular degeneration). This is a disorder of lipid metabolism in which an abnormal deposition of fat in the organs can be demonstrated in infants. Blindness, mental deterioration and convulsions may result. There is a strong tendency for this disease to occur in some families, especially Jewish.

The metabolic disorders presented here are only a few characteristic examples. Many more are known or may be detected in the near future.

B. TOXIC DISORDERS

1. Alcohol (ethyl; C_2H_5OH). This agent can probably damage any part of the nervous system. In *Wernicke's encephalopathy* the areas around the third ventricle and the mammillary bodies show degeneration. Frequently *Korsakoff's psychosis* can develop: the patient has visual hallucinations and feels persecuted and threatened by strange-looking animals. Major personality changes occur and the patient imagines things like snakes, rats, dogs, cats, etc. all about him in the room.

The *corpus callosum* can be affected by Italian red wine, which can cause interference with impulses between the two hemispheres (Marchiafava-Bignami disease). Frequently the *cerebellum* is affected and the Purkinje cell layer reveals atrophy. The *pons* may be involved, in cases of central pontine myelinolysis. Most frequently the peripheral nerves, *especially the sensory fibers*, get involved, and the neuropathy due to alcohol is more painful than that in diabetes (squeezing of the calf muscles causes pain). In all of these entities, especially in Wernicke's disease, the quick administration of vitamin B_1 is important.

2. Methyl alcohol. This chemical substance has an affinity for the optic nerve (II) and causes blindness. After the acute episode affecting the optic nerve, a long-range involvement of the putamen, with extrapyramidal tract symptoms, may occur. The damage to the optic nerve is caused by acetaldehyde, which has a special affinity for the nerve fibers. Frequently the methanol, or "wood alcohol", is consumed by mistake because of improper labelling of bottles or illicit manufacture of liquors. Depending on the amount of intake, complete blindness can sometimes be prevented.

3. Lead poisoning. This heavy metal can produce an encephalopathy with frequent seizures. It may be fatal, especially in children who pick up the lead content in paint, particularly from painted wooden toys, cribs, high chairs, etc. It is important to determine the lead level of the blood, which should not be more than 40 micrograms/ml.

The treatment of lead poisoning is with chelating agents such as Penicillamine, which combines with lead and eliminates it from the body in the urine. Inhalation of exhaust fumes from cars using leaded gasoline can also be a causative factor in children. Increased blood levels of lead are found in workers in battery factories. Frequently a radial nerve palsy results, with the characteristic "wrist drop." Just why lead attacks the radial nerve before other peripheral nerves is not known.

4. Other metals. Magnesium, mercury and gold, for example, can cause similar symptoms to those of lead poisoning.

5. Disease processes. Certain diseases, such as diphtheria and food poisoning (botulism), can produce endotoxins which cause nervous system paralysis. The paralysis with diphtheria usually starts in the lower extremities, extending later on to the trunk and upper extremities. Treatment is by the use of antitoxins and the symptoms may resolve in the reverse order.

Chapter 9

PERIPHERAL NEUROPATHIES

It should be understood at the outset that there are different kinds of nerve fibers, all with certain characteristics. Conduction velocity is related to the diameter of the fiber; the larger the fiber, the faster the speed of conduction.

Group A Fibers These are myelinated and are 1–20 microns in diameter. They carry touch and pressure sensations and conduct at a velocity of 30–100 meters/sec.

Group B Fibers These are myelinated and are only 3 microns in diameter. They carry pain and temperature sensations and conduct at a maximum velocity of 10 meters/sec.

Group C Fibers These are unmyelinated and have a diameter of only 1 micron. They carry diffuse pain and efferent vasomotor impulses and conduct at a velocity of 1–2 meters/sec.

In Wallerian degeneration, the distal part of the nerve peripheral to the area of trauma degenerates. Regeneration after trauma to the nerve may result in neuroma formation. Seventy percent of the fibers usually grow into the peripheral end (broadly speaking, through the neurilemmal cords), and reestablish contact with the structure originally supplied; up to thirty percent of the fibers may produce the painful, tumor-like neuroma. In the peripheral nervous system, the severed nerve fiber grows at a rate of 1–2 mm. per day. If a nerve has been completely severed, the nerve ends may have to be approximated surgically and interspersed fragments of bone removed. Occasionally a hematoma develops at the trauma site and has to be removed.

Neuropraxia is defined as external compression or injury to a nerve, without degeneration, followed by rapid and complete recovery of function. *Axonotmesis* is a crushing injury which destroys the continuity of the axon without damage to the supporting tissues. *Neurotmesis* is severance of an entire nerve. Nerve fibers in the central nervous system (brain and spinal cord) do not regenerate as do those in the peripheral nerves, as far as we know.

A. DIFFUSE NEUROPATHIES

Most of these are due to degenerative changes in the peripheral nerves. The term "neuritis" should be reserved for peripheral nerve involvement due to tuberculosis or syphilis, which cause an actual inflammation of the nerves.

1. Toxic agents (especially metals). As mentioned before, lead intoxication may cause radial nerve paralysis and subsequent wrist drop. With arsenic, gold and mercury the neuropathy involves the sensory fibers first and then the motor fibers.

2. Organic agents. Carbon monoxide poisoning may cause involvement of both the sensory and motor fibers. The skin usually shows a cherry-red color.

3. Immune sera. Frequently given in early life, these often affect the nerves in the region of the brachial plexus.

4. Deficiency states and metabolic disorders (see also chapter 8).

a) Chronic alcoholism.   The condition usually affects the sensory fibers first. The lower extremities are involved earlier than the upper. As previously mentioned this symptom is probably due to a vitamin B_1 deficiency. In severe cases patients may show the picture of *pseudotabes alcoholica*, in which not only the peripheral nerves are involved but the posterior columns of the spinal cord are also slightly affected.

b) Diabetes mellitus.   Again, the sensory fibers in the feet are affected first; later on there is motor involvement. In severe cases a *pseudotabes diabetica* may result with the posterior columns affected as in chronic alcoholism. A femoral neuropathy is occasionally encountered (more so in diabetes than in any other disease. Other causes of femoral neuropathy are metastatic carcinoma and bleeding into the nerve sheath in cases of anticoagulant therapy.)

c) Porphyria (see page 82).

d) Infections

    i. *Diphtheria* is an ascending neuropathy starting in the lower extremities. If it reaches the level of C_4 it may result in paralysis of the diaphragm and the patient may need artificial respiration.

    ii. *Infectious Mononucleosis* is a condition in which the facial nerve (VII) is frequently affected (see mononeuropathies, page 89).

    iii. *Sarcoidosis* (*Boeck*).   Exhibits basilar meningeal proliferations, which can be diffuse or focal. Not infrequently there is a bilateral facial nerve palsy. Infiltration of nerve roots and peripheral nerves also occurs.

    iv. *Hansen's Disease* (*leprosy*) may cause a severe type of peripheral neuropathy. This entity is a bacterial disease caused by Mycobacterium leprae and is extremely rare in the United States; the highest incidence is in tropical climates.

e) Vascular disease.   In cases of arteriosclerosis the peripheral nerves may be affected by way of the vasa nervorum, due to lack of oxygenation. A few patients may have an inflammation of the blood vessel wall (vasculitis) which reduces the blood flow by narrowing the lumen.

f) Guillain-Barré syndrome.   This is a type of infectious neuropathy, described first in the trenches of World War I, with segmental demyelination of the peripheral nerves; it may be due to an unknown virus. Usually it affects motor fibers at the anterior root level first, but can also affect the sensory fibers. Weakness of the extremities, especially the lower ones, is noted. The thigh muscles are chiefly affected, and deep tendon reflexes are diminished or absent.

It is seen these days especially in individuals who work in low-temperature areas such as breweries, packing plants, etc.; it is also found as a complication of flu innoculations. It occurs more frequently during the colder seasons of the year. A spinal tap done approximately two to three days after the onset will reveal an increasing high protein content but no cells (dissociation of albumen and cells). The mortality rate used to be very high, but is now reduced to about 10% or less. A respirator should always be kept at hand because the disease tends to ascend and involve the arms, diaphragm and brain stem as well. Early and intensive physical therapy with active and passive exercises is of paramount importance.

B. MONONEUROPATHIES

1. Facial palsy (Bell). Probably the most frequent neuropathy affecting a cranial nerve. This is a condition of unknown etiology but may be of a viral type. The facial nerve usually swells up in the facial canal producing pain in the area of the ear and paralysis. It tends to be one-sided, occurring more on the side exposed to draft and cold winds (i.e., air conditioners).

All branches of the nerve are equally affected (lower motor neurons), unlike facial palsies in strokes or tumors, where only the two lower branches of the facial nerve (upper motor neurons) are involved. The danger of a corneal ulcer exists because of the inability to close the eye and keep it moist. Eighty percent of the patients improve to almost normal; twenty percent do not improve completely and may require face-lifts later on.

Electromyography and nerve conduction studies will help to determine the prognosis; these are usually done after the second or third day. A slight delay in motor conduction time only is favorable, while no response by electrical stimulation is an unfavorable sign. The normal conduction time from the point of stimulus at the stylomastoid foramen to the orbicularis oris or oculi is approximately 4.0 msec. The nerve conduction time to these muscles and to the frontalis is determined, and the seventh nerve threshold is also determined (usually higher on the involved side).

In the treatment of this condition daily muscle exercises in front of a mirror are beneficial. Electrical stimulations of the nerve fibers should be done only once or twice each week, in order to prevent contractures later on. Only in rare instances is it necessary to decompress the nerve surgically in the facial canal.

Improvement usually occurs over a period of three to six months. Since the patient cannot wrinkle the forehead or close the eyes, the eyes should be looked after at regular intervals; at times an eye patch may be necessary.

Face-lift procedures are done chiefly for their cosmetic value, especially in women. The facial nerve may be *bilaterally* involved in sarcoidosis (page 88), and in Recklinghausen's disease (neurofibromatosis); where cerebello-pontine angle neuromas may also produce bilateral involvement.

2. Carpal tunnel syndrome. This is the most important entrapment syndrome and involves the median nerve, because of its compression by the transverse carpal ligament. The syndrome occurs frequently in obesity, pregnancy, arthritis, trauma to the wrist and amyloidosis. All of these entities cause swelling and narrowing of the carpal tunnel. The first symptom is a pinprick feeling, with loss of sensitivity, in the thumb, index and middle fingers and the radial half of the ring finger, accompanied by pain in the wrist region.

Much later, atrophy of the opponens pollicis muscle develops. Percussion over the median nerve will cause a tingling sensation which radiates into the fingers (Tinel sign), indicating a partial lesion or beginning regeneration.

The syndrome is often bilateral but usually more pronounced in the dominant hand. After initial cortisone injections (which are usually only of intermittent help) the treatment consists of surgically cutting the transverse carpal ligament and freeing the underlying nerve (neurolysis); the surgery is effective in nine out of ten cases.

The median nerve can also be entrapped at the site of the pronator teres muscle. This may occur in people active in sports such as volleyball, etc., and in those using frequent pronation and supination of the forearm. Again, cortisone injections are of help. Occasionally surgical intervention will be necessary in order to eliminate possible calcification of the muscle.

3. Ulnar nerve. Compression of this nerve against the medial epicondyle of the humerus is a frequent cause of inability to adduct or abduct the fingers (interossei musculature). On occasion, the nerve may be dislocated at the epicondyle, and surgical procedures may be necessary to relocate the nerve into the normal bony canal.

4. Radial nerve. Usually affected in fractures of the middle part of the humerus. Since the nerve is very close to the underlying bone, fragments of bony splinters should be looked for. In manipulating the bone to approximate the opposing ends for setting (following fractures, during surgical procedures), care must be exercised to prevent damage to the nerve by the jagged bone ends.

5. Common peroneal nerve. Frequently involved in compression of the nerve against the head of the fibula. This may occur by the application of knee bandages which are too tight and by prolonged kneeling. The result is foot drop and a "stork-like" gait; inspection of footwear will reveal excessive wearing of the sole at the tip. Neurologic examination of this lesion may also demonstrate a possible sensory loss. Loosening of the bandage will alleviate the condition when it's due to bandage tightness.

6. Tarsal tunnel syndrome. The tibial nerve in its passage around the medial malleolus may be compressed by the flexor retinaculum (laciniate ligament). The compression may also be due to the swelling of varicose veins, obesity, and tight footwear, and may be seen in malformed feet. The patient has pain and numbness in the sole of the foot and weakness of the intrinsic foot muscles. Cortisone injections or surgical intervention may be required. The syndrome is diagnosed by EMG and nerve conduction studies. It is much less frequent than the carpal tunnel syndrome described previously.

7. Erb's palsy. A lesion of the brachial plexus which mainly involves nerve roots C_5 and C_6 and the proximal arm musculature (biceps, brachioradialis, deltoid, etc.). The condition may be due to a high forceps delivery at birth, or to a severe fall on the outstretched arm.

8. Klumpke's paralysis. A condition which involves the brachial plexus at the levels of C_8 and T_1 affecting mainly the intrinsic muscles of the hand and flexors of the wrist and fingers. It may result from a severe fall on the outstretched hand.

In serious injuries, not infrequently a complete brachial plexus paralysis may result (gunshot and stab wounds, etc.). Occasionally hematomas develop in the brachial plexus region and may have to be removed surgically.

Rehabilitation procedures should be aimed at prevention of "freezing" of the joints and muscular wasting until the nerve-muscle contact is restored. This is usually done by passive and, later on, active exercises, as well as by massage or heat treatment. A minor degree of muscular atrophy due to inactivity cannot always be prevented. Splinting of the affected limb may have to be done during the recovery period.

Chapter 10

INTERVERTEBRAL DISK HERNIATIONS AND TRAUMATIC CORD INJURIES

The cause of intervertebral disk herniation in almost every instance is acute or chronic trauma. Each disk is composed of a peripheral portion of fibrous tissue and fibro-cartilage, the *annulus fibrosus*, and a central soft, pulpy, elastic substance, the *nucleus pulposus* (a remnant of the notochord) (Fig. 16). Severe strain or trauma causes the disk to protrude beyond its normal limits, the annulus fibrosus is torn and the nucleus pulposus herniates out against the adjacent nerve root.

At the cervical and lumbar levels herniations rarely occur anteriorly into the neck or abdomen, because the anterior longitudinal ligament is considerably stronger than the posterior ligament (Fig. 17). The posterior longitudinal ligament is especially weak in the lateral regions, hence most disks protrude posteriorly and laterally. Ninety percent of disk prolapses occur at the level of L_3-L_4 and L_4-L_5. Eight percent occur in the cervical area and only two percent in the thoracic region. In the latter, herniations are usually associated with diseases such as tuberculosis or osteo-myelitis. Degenerative changes in older people contribute to this occurrence, which may then be precipitated by mild trauma. In rare cases inflammatory diseases of the disks are the cause.

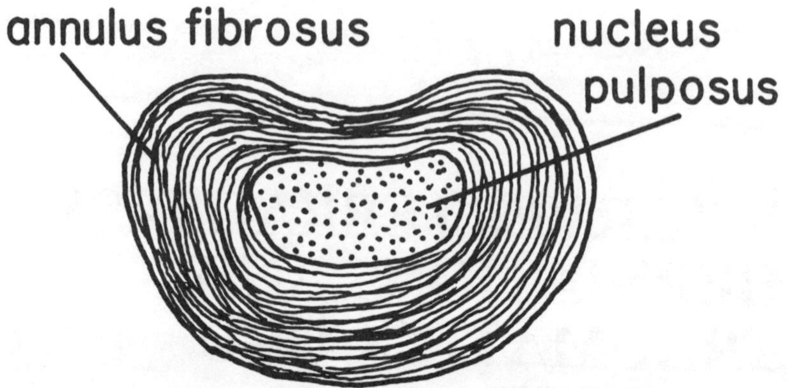

Figure 16. Diagram of transverse section of an intervertebral disk. Note that the nucleus pulposus tends to be located somewhat posteriorly.

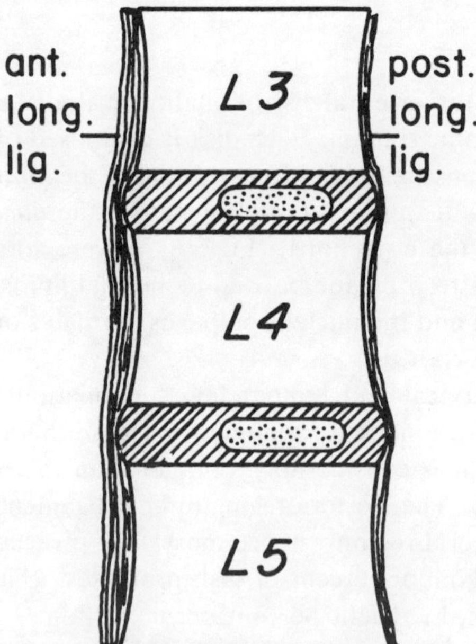

Figure 17. Diagram of a midsagittal section through the third, fourth and fifth lumbar vertebrae showing the relative thickness of the anterior compared to the posterior longitudinal ligaments.

Disk degenerations were described as early as 1857 by Virchow. It was not until 1934, when radiopaque material was used, that intervertebral disks could be demonstrated exerting pressure on one or more nerve roots (myelography) or on the spinal cord. The incidence of herniation is greater in men than in women.

In *lumbar disk herniations* there is usually severe pain in the back of the thigh radiating into the posterior part of the leg. The ankle jerk reflex tends to be diminished or absent. The root pain is usually in the gluteal region and radiates down the sciatic nerve; it is aggravated by coughing, sneezing, straining and body movements. The pain is usually of intermittent type and there is considerable additional muscle spasm which limits movements. One-fourth of the patients have pain at night and they are uncomfortable in bed; walking and sitting may bring relief.

Disk problems are the most frequent causes of low back pain, besides spasms of the lumbar musculature due to strain. A careful history and neurologic examination are essential. Frequently, chronic trauma will bring on a slowly progressing symptomatology. The *first* symptoms are usually due to *irritation* and cause lower back pain. The lumbar curvature is less pronounced than normal, there are spasms of the spinal musculature and a tilting of the trunk away from the lesion to ease the pain caused by the nerve root being compressed against the bone. If there is a midline disk developing, the patient may demonstrate a "corkscrew" type of motion in order to diminish the pain. This stage usually causes partial disability and is helped by bed rest, local application of heat, light massage and placing a board underneath the mattress. Muscle relaxants such as Robaxin, Valium or Dantrium may be of help.

If the problems do not improve, the *second stage, compression*, may be reached. The nerve roots are compressed during coughing, sneezing or bowel movements. Paresthesia develops at the outer aspect of the calf musculature, foot and toes; local tenderness can be observed. The Lasègue phenomenon (in which the leg is elevated) will cause pain in the lumbar region, either unilateral or (sometimes) bilateral. The patient cannot sit up without pain. The ankle jerk reflex is usually absent if the nerve root at L_5 is involved. Conservative treatment can still be attempted, but if the patient does not improve in three to four weeks, myelography and surgical intervention may become necessary. This is especially true if the patient has already had several bouts of sciatic pain previously.

The *third stage, paresis*, may be reached, in which the patient is considerably disabled. He develops weakness of the foot musculature as well as atrophy; usually peroneal muscle weakness results. A sensory deficit is present and the ankle reflex is absent. If the lesion is at a higher lumbar level, the knee reflex may be impaired.

The *fourth stage, paralysis*, occurs if several roots are involved or the spinal cord itself is compressed at higher levels. Bladder and bowel disturbances occur if the lesion is above the level of L_2 (sacral cord compression). Treatment consists of urgent operative interference by laminectomy. As indicated before, the diagnosis is made by myelography, although, on occasion, plain X-rays of the lumbar spine may show the narrowed intervertebral space.

The spinal fluid in these cases reveals an increase of protein below the massive disk prolapse. In certain cases there is recurrence of the symptoms, especially if the disability occurred during work. A differential diagnosis, especially in older people, should be made to rule out cancer metastases, which usually involve the vertebral bodies rather than the disk space. Disk disease, together with low back pain, is probably the most abused entity among people trying to get compensation benefits. In these cases the condition may "never" improve.

There is a direct relation between the size of the vertebral canal and the symptoms of disk herniation at the lumbar and cervical levels. In patients with small vertebral canals disk symptoms are more frequent and appear much earlier than in others. *Cervical disk herniation* is considerably less frequent than lumbar protrusions. They are usually in the midline and may compress the spinal cord; chiefly involved here is the lower cervical area (C_5-C_8). Root pain radiating into the arms results, although it is possible, on occasion, that no pain is manifest. Straightening of the neck curvature may occur and motions of the neck are painful; the muscles will reveal spasms. Biceps, supinator or triceps reflexes may be interfered with. Hypalgesia in certain dermatomes may occur. If the pain is in the thumb and index finger the root at C_6 is involved, while at C_7 the middle finger is affected; the lesion at

C_8 will involve the ring and little fingers. In cervical disk degeneration the wearing of a soft collar or neck traction, usually starting with 7–10 pounds over several weeks, may be of help. Surgical intervention by laminectomy after several weeks of consecutive therapy may have to be resorted to. *Thoracic disks* are much less common and usually protrude in the midline posteriorly.

Spondylolisthesis is a forward displacement of one vertebra over another.

Severe *compression of the spinal cord* due to trauma for more than 10–15 minutes usually results in loss of function and irreparable damage. A cord injury at the level of C_1-C_2 is usually fatal. If the odontoid process of the axis is fractured, the head may be tilted and stiff, resulting in damage to the underlying medulla oblongata. A cord injury at the levels of C_3, C_4 and C_5 causes respiratory paralysis due to involvement of the diaphragm (phrenic nerve). The forearms are usually kept flexed and the arms are rotated outward. With injuries at the C_6-C_7 level the forearms are usually flexed and lying on the chest. Safe transportation of the patient is essential and prompt surgical treatment is needed. If the spinal cord is damaged and sensory loss results, any pressure upon the skin should be prevented, and developing decubiti should be treated at once. *Unskillful lifting* of the patient can cause a complete transection of the spinal cord! Although prompt surgical attention is essential in these cases, it frequently comes too late, because of the time lost in transporting the patient to the hospital.

Chapter 11

DEMYELINATING AND DEGENERATIVE DISEASES

A. DEMYELINATING DISEASES

1. Multiple sclerosis (MS, disseminated sclerosis or polysclerosis).
This disease was described by Cruveilhier in France in 1835 and subsequently by Carswell in Great Britain in 1838. This is an entity of unknown etiology, with remissions and relapses due to patches of demyelination followed by sclerosis in the brain, spinal cord and, rarely, in the peripheral nervous system. The classic hallmark for this disease is *Charcot's Triad*:

- Ataxia.
- Nystagmus.
- Scanning (spastic) speech.

Multiple sclerosis affects all races and all regions of the world. However, it is prevalent in the northern European countries (Norway and Sweden) and in Canada. The incidence in northern Europe reaches 3 per 1000 population; in central Europe the figure is lower, being about 1 per 1000. In the northern United States incidence is higher than in the southern states. The disease is less frequent in the area around the Mediterranean Sea, and there is a considerably lower incidence in Asia and Africa.

Eighty percent of the cases have their onset between the ages of 20–40 years. Ten percent start before the age of 20 and ten percent between the ages of 40–55. Rare cases are described in children, and females are affected slightly more than males. The most prevalent theory at the present time is that multiple sclerosis may be an autoimmune disease or a disease caused by a slow virus.

If the slow virus theory is correct, the patient may acquire the infection as a teenager and may harbor the virus for several years before the disease manifests itself. Exposure to a cold and damp climate may precipitate the illness. Demyelinating disease has been produced in animals but this is not strictly comparable with the multiple sclerosis observed in humans.

Many theories about the origin have been put forward: microbic invasion, small venous thrombi, allergic and antigenic responses, as well as involvement of the perivascular lymphatic channels and blood vessels. Pathologically the demyelinated areas are well outlined and assume all kinds of shapes and sizes, usually scattered throughout the white matter of the central nervous system. In the beginning the areas are usually pinkish with lymphocytic infiltration.

The demyelinating process destroys fat and produces some kind of neutral fat which accumulates around the blood vessels and is then absorbed by the blood stream and transported away. The myelin destruction occurs in three stages:

1. Destruction of a circumscribed area and production of neutral fat.

2. Accumulation of perivascular lipids and then gradual disappearance of the fat.

3. Infiltration of glial cells, which make the area grayish in color and harder than the surrounding regions. The plaque may extend into the gray matter of the brain and cord.

In the acute stage of lymphocytic infiltration (when the plaques are pinkish) some edema develops around the demyelinating process. This subsides after the acute stage and

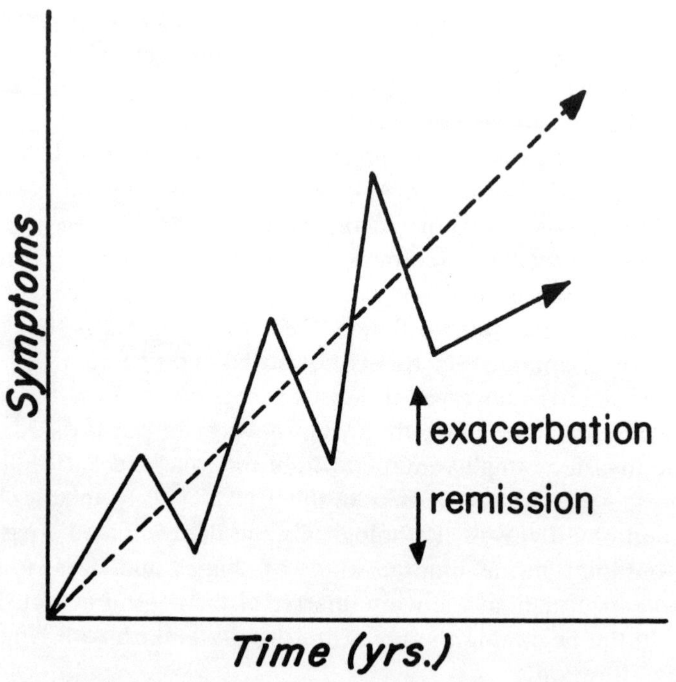

Figure 18.   Profile of multiple sclerosis showing exacerbations and remissions characteristic of the disease (solid arrow), with steady progression of different symptoms (broken arrow).

accounts for the remissions in this disease. Plaques in the brain may encroach upon the cortex and produce epileptic seizures in five percent of cases. Pathologically the myelin sheaths of the nerve fibers are destroyed and the axis cylinders are exposed; the axis cylinder is affected only to a minor degree.

Anatomical areas frequently involved are regions around the lateral ventricles, the aqueduct and the optic nerve. Frequently the demyelinated areas center around arteries and veins. In the spinal cord they tend to be slightly more irregular and rarely encroach upon the gray matter.

Clinically the disease can start at any place, but usually when it occurs (in the early twenties) the optic nerves are affected first. There is evidence of papillitis (usually unilateral) for ten days to three weeks. Later, temporal pallor of the optic disk may result, after the swelling subsides and vision (which has been partially obscured) improves.

The papillo-macular bundle may be affected and the patient may have unilateral retrobulbar neuritis, which is even more common than the above-described papillitis. In this case, retro-orbital pain develops, and again temporal pallor of the optic disk may result. No changes of the optic disk, as seen by fundoscopy, can be noticed in the beginning.

In many cases the contralateral eye becomes involved in the same way six months to one year later. If the papillo-macular bundle is affected, the central vision may be impaired and a central scotoma, on visual field examination, may develop. Just why the papillo-macular bundle is particularly vulnerable to demyelination is not known.

From now on the disease may stop at any time but in most cases, unfortunately, it progresses slowly with remissions and exacerbations (Fig. 18). Multiple sclerosis has been called the "chameleon" of neurologic diseases, because it can imitate almost all syndromes.

The next finding may be nystagmus. It is interesting to note that the abducting eye is affected more than the adducting eye in horizontal movement. Some cases may also develop vertical or even rotatory nystagmus. Due to abducens nerve palsy, double vison in the horizontal plane may manifest itself.

Frequently the cerebellum is involved and there is marked ataxia in the upper extremities, with intention tremor. If the patient is asked to touch his nose with his index finger, a marked tremor will develop as the finger approaches the nose (finger-nose test). The patient also walks with an ataxic gait and has difficulty in keeping his balance. Usually the upper extremities show more pronounced cerebellar involvement than the lower.

Progression of the disease results in pyramidal tract symptoms with marked spasticity, which is usually more intense in the legs than in the arms. Pronounced Babinski phenomena can be elicited and abdominal reflexes are lost early. The disease rarely progresses symmetrically; the symptoms are, for the most part, asymmetrical. The posterior columns may become involved and vibratory sense will then be decreased in the extremities.

Other symptoms may include a neurogenic spastic bladder with difficulty starting urination, or with an atonic bladder, in which case there is difficulty in holding the urine. Bladder and kidney complications are commonly introduced by the prolonged use of catheters, and an ascending pyelonephritis (E. coli infection) may develop. These infections should be controlled by antibiotic therapy.

If the lesion is around the third ventricle, a euphoria (elevated mood) of the patient is rather characteristic. The patient probably lacks insight into the condition and, in spite of the seriousness of the disease, is in good spirits. One "philosopher" suggested that it might be God's way of compensating. Occasionally, though, a patient with MS may be depressed.

The life span of the MS patient is somewhat reduced (by approximately ten years), although the survival rate during the past decade has been improving. This may be due to less severe demyelinating processes occurring at the present time or it may be due to better treatment. Characteristic symptoms may occur with a plaque in the cervical cord close to the meninges. In this case bending the neck produces a severe "electrical shock," with pain going down the spine. This is the "electrical sign of Lhermitte."

Clinical varieties of the disease include forms which affect only the spinal cord, the cerebrum, the cerebellum or the pons. Rarely is the amyotrophic form of MS seen in which there is atrophy of the intrinsic muscles of the hand. Personal and behavioral changes do occur and there is a considerable range of emotions to be noticed.

If both hemispheres have demyelinating processes, pathologic laughter or crying may develop (the patient starts to laugh or cry for no reason and has difficulty stopping). Defects in intelligence, due to lesions in the frontal and temporal lobes, occur relatively late in the disease. During its prolonged course, the patient usually becomes confined to a wheelchair or bedridden for many years.

Rarer forms of multiple sclerosis exist and include:

Hemiplegic type found in female teenagers. The picture is similar to a stroke but the weakness of one side of the body occurs over a period of three to four days instead of minutes or hours. This is due to an extensive demyelinating process in the contralateral hemisphere. Although studies such as arteriography or myelography should be kept to a minimum in MS, arteriographic studies and CT-scan in such a special case are necessary to rule out a rapidly growing brain tumor. Repeated spinal taps may exacerbate the disease and cause a new bout of demyelination.

Paraparetic form. This is a type of MS which occurs in women usually beyond the age of 40–50 years in which there is demyelination in the middle and lower spinal cord. There are marked motor and sensory symptoms below the level of the lesion. The usual remissions and exacerbations are not found and the condition deteriorates rather gradually. A myelogram has to be done, even though the procedure may temporarily aggravate the process, to rule out a spinal cord tumor, which may produce the same symptoms. In very rare cases a spinal cord tumor (lipoma or fibroma) may be present in patients with demyelinating conditions.

Pregnancy can also exacerbate the symptoms of multiple sclerosis and many people feel that an abortion should be done during the first three months of gestation. However, spinal anesthesia should be avoided in all cases of MS! During the acute stage of the demyelinating process, lymphocytes may be found in the spinal fluid. There may also be some polymorphonuclear leukocytes; usually 20–50 white blood cells are found per cu. mm.

The normal protein content of the spinal fluid is 30–40 mg% but in MS it is frequently above 50 mg%, although below 100 mg% in the majority of cases. Electrophoresis of the spinal fluid shows elevation of gamma globulins but, again, this is not specific, since it may also occur in tumors and syphilis.

The treatment of this disease is difficult to evaluate because of the remission of symptoms. Massage and muscle relaxants such as Valium, Robaxin or Dantrium can be used to ease the muscular spasticity and to loosen the musculature. Cold and damp weather should be avoided; the patients will usually feel better in warm and dry climates, which may lessen the progress of the disease to some degree. Animal fat should be avoided and replaced by un-saturated fat. Physical and occupational therapy are of great importance in this disease, although the benefit is difficult to estab-lish.

In rare cases the demyelinating process takes on a fulminating aspect and a patient may die within a few years, usually due to an aspiration pneumonia. Bladder symptoms should be carefully looked for throughout the course of this situation to avoid any ascending urinary infection. The patient should also be checked for decubiti, which will develop especially in areas where there is some loss of sensation (buttocks and ankle regions in particular).

2. Schilder's disease (Diffuse sclerosis). This is a more widespread sclerosis and a rapidly progressive illness. Large areas of demye-lination occur in the white matter of both hemispheres, especially in the parietal and occipital regions. The disease usually starts in young children after they have had a normal infancy and early childhood. Within a year or two the disease has usually progressed to complete blindness, dementia and marked spasticity. The dis-ease progresses steadily and remissions do not occur.

An internal compensatory hydrocephalus may develop, as-sociated with a massive destruction, especially of the subcortical white matter, causing cavitation. The cerebellum, pons and spinal cord are usually spared and the gray matter is not often involved. A marked microglial and astrocytic infiltration of the demyelinated areas occurs, and slight meningeal reactions have been found.

More often than not, mood changes are observed in these children at school. They become more quiet and their intellectual activity is somewhat blunted. Nausea and vomiting may occur, as well as convulsions, and the wandering eye movements of blindness can be noticed. Optic atrophy will be found. Vision is usually lost before walking becomes impossible due to the marked spasticity. Speech difficulties can occur, hearing may fail and decerebrate rigidity may become manifest. Death usually ensues after a few months, the maximum survival time being 4–5 years. There is no known specific therapy; prevention of infection and regular feeding are most important.

3. Krabbe's disease. This is a diffuse sclerosis which starts in the first year of life. It leads to marked spasticity, convulsions and loss of vision. The patient may also show decerebrate rigidity, deafness, blindness and frequent seizures.

4. Neuromyelitis optica (Devic's disease). This is probably a subform of multiple sclerosis which is frequently found in the young. It affects the optic nerves and causes pallor and atrophy of the entire optic disk, usually bilaterally. This is frequently followed by an infectious process in the spinal cord occurring at the thoracic level most of the time. Numbness and tingling as well as paralysis of the musculature can be found below the level of the lesion. This is called a *transverse myelitis*. The process is self-limited, for the most part, and progresses only occasionally.

The chief clinical symptoms are a rapid loss of vision of one eye, followed by the same process on the opposite side. On occasion a mild upper respiratory infection may be present. The visual loss is more sudden than in the common form of multiple sclerosis. Within a few days or weeks after the eye findings, a meningeal irritation may occur, with weakness and paresthesias of the lower part of the body. Spontaneous resolution usually occurs within a few weeks, although the optic atrophy persists and brisk reflexes commonly remain in the lower extremities. Rarely does the disease start with a transverse myelitis followed by optic neuritis. After recovery there is usually no recurrence (80–90%). The spinal tap reveals 50–100 cells/ml. in the acute stage and the protein is two to three times the normal amount.

5. Leber's optic atrophy. This is a sex-linked, recessive condition which affects only males. The disease occurs around the time of puberty and up to age 25. The patient may complain of hazy vision and pain in his eye. A central scotoma may develop and there may be loss of central vision in both eyes, although occasionally only one eye is involved. No other neurologic signs can be observed. Again, the demyelination most markedly affects the papillo-macular bundle. In cases of optic atrophy, a syphilitic infection or a tumor of the hypophysis should be ruled out.

B. DEGENERATIVE DISEASES

1. Cerebellar Diseases

a) Primary. An example of this is *Friedreich's Ataxia* which is relatively rare and autosomal recessively inherited. The spinal cord is affected, and the lateral and posterior columns as well as both spinocerebellar tracts are involved. The process usually starts between the ages of 10–20 years. The hallmarks of this entity are high-arched feet and marked ataxia. The knee and ankle reflexes are usually absent. The disease progresses very slowly. *This is the most important example of the many degenerative cerebellar diseases which occur.* There may be as many as fifty different types.

b) Secondary. These usually cause Purkinje cell degeneration, as with alcohol, carcinoma and anoxia. Dilantin can also adversely affect the cerebellum.

2. Amyotrophic Lateral Sclerosis (ALS)

The etiology of this disease is unknown and there is no specific medication available. It usually strikes in the fifth decade and affects males slightly more than females. Juvenile forms of the disease have been described but are rare. ALS is usually relentlessly progressive, with death ensuing in a period of 18 months to 10 years. The Betz cells of the cerebral cortex, the pyramidal tract in the brain stem and spinal cord, and the anterior horn cells are affected. The disease may start at the lower or upper motor neuron level. If the lower motor neurons are affected, the muscular loss is seen earliest and best in the hand. Should the disease start in the anterior horn cells and progress slowly upward, the life expectancy may be as long as 8–10 years. If the disease starts at the brain stem level, affecting the cranial nerve nuclei (especially XII) it may result in tongue atrophy with fasciculations (see pages 9, 67).

Life expectancy with brain stem involvement is only one to two years, with the patients usually dying of complications such as pneumonia. Clinical observations will most frequently disclose weakness and atrophy of the interossei musculature, and occasionally the peroneal muscles are wasted. Marked spasticity, usually combined with atrophy of the muscles and weight loss, sets in; the patient gradually becomes bedridden. While no specific medication is known, physical therapy may be of some help, especially in the early stages, to overcome the spasticity. Although research is continuing, the cause of ALS has yet to be found.

3. Syringomyelia

This is a disease affecting the spinal cord; if the brain stem is involved, the condition is called *syringobulbia*. It usually occurs in the cervical region of the spinal cord with paracentral cavitation (Fig. 19). It may block the reflex arcs in the upper extremities and show diminished or absent reflexes at the level of the syrinx. Below the level of the cavitation, pyramidal tract findings are abundant, with increased reflexes and spasticity of the legs.

The hallmark of this disease is loss of the modalities of *pain and temperature* (contralateral to the cord lesion) resulting in patients frequently burning themselves (by cigarettes, stoves, etc.) because they cannot feel the heat. This sensory loss is due to the involvement of the lateral spinothalamic tract fibers, which are interrupted by the cavitation. Patients also have difficulty sensing cold. If the syrinx extends forward the anterior horn cells become involved.

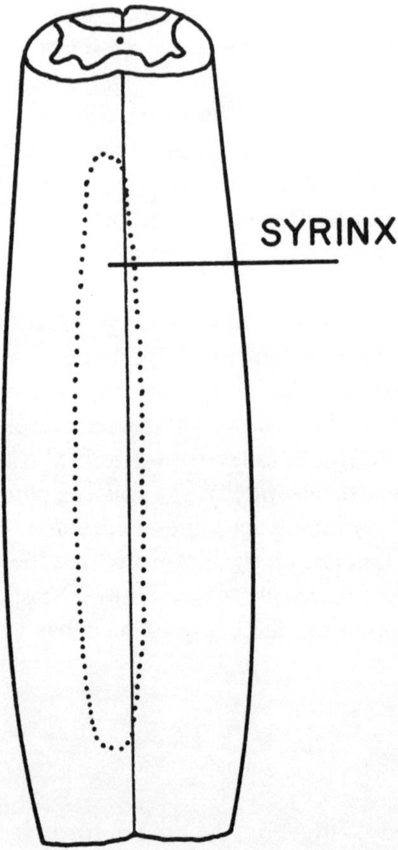

Figure 19.   Diagram of a longitudinal view of the spinal cord showing the outline of the paracentral cavitation in syringomyelia and the accompanying cord enlargement. Note that the syrinx tends to lie to one side of the midline.

At the area of the cavitation there may be an enlargement of the spinal cord, which can be found by myelography; in 50% of the cases the diagnosis can be established this way. The disease tends to start between ages 10 and 20 and more often than not in persons who have other physical malformations, such as kyphosis, scoliosis, cleft palate or spina bifida occulta. The disease progresses relatively slowly. If the cranial nerve nuclei in the brain stem are involved (especially the hypoglossal nerve), there is difficulty with chewing and swallowing. After the diagnosis is established, X-ray treatment of the cavitation may be of some help in avoiding enlargement of the syrinx. Surgical exploration may have to be done for the purpose of draining the cavitation.

4. Pre-Senile Dementias

These occur in the 55 to 70-year-old group. Since the life span in this country is increasing, these dementias have been making their appearance somewhat later than they did 20 to 30 years ago, when they occurred between the ages of 50–60 years.

a) Alzheimer's disease. Atrophy of the cerebral cortex, which occurs gradually and affects the parietal or occipital areas in particular. Signs of declining intelligence and psychologic testing will give evidence of organic brain disease (performance will be more impaired than verbal IQ). A CT-scan will clearly show the wasting of the cortex (pneumoencephalography is rarely done today). Occasionally a patient with Alzheimer's disease may develop epileptic seizures which can be observed clinically and verified by the electroencephalogram.

b) Pick's disease. This is a more localized atrophic condition which affects the frontal and temporal regions in particular. The patient neglects his body, jokes inappropriately and shows a lack of awareness of other people. He may have difficulty walking (astasia) or standing (abasia), and the condition usually leads to complete dementia.

These patients do not have epileptic seizures and do not decline as rapidly in mental function as those with Alzheimer's disease (CT-scan will demonstrate the focal cortical atrophy). Patients with either of these dementias usually have to be placed into mental institutions.

c) Jakob-Creutzfeldt disease. A rare condition with gradually developing dementia. Cells in the gray matter of the brain and spinal cord are degenerated. These patients have associated extrapyr-amidal signs, as evidenced by a fixed facial expression and Par-kinsonian tremor.

Myoclonic jerks and seizures may accompany the symptoms. The end result of this process is a profoundly demented, wasted, aphasic and rigid patient. The EEG usually shows generalized, progressively increasing, slowing or repetitive epileptiform dis-charges. The CT-scan reveals cortical atrophy, cerebellar wasting and a ventricular dilation.

The diagnoses of the three above diseases can be made by cortical biopsies and, in the case of Jakob-Creutzfeldt disease, by demonstration of a slow-virus.

Chapter 12

TUMORS OF THE BRAIN AND SPINAL CORD

9% of all body tumors are located within the central nervous system. Of these, 80% are in the brain and 20% are in the spinal cord.

A. BRAIN TUMORS

Symptoms

1. Headache usually on the side of the tumor; this may awaken the patient at night (see Fig. 13, Profile 6).

2. Seizures are more apt to be unilateral (contralateral to the lesion) but are occasionally generalized. This is especially important in the absence of a previous history of epilepsy. Approximately 20–30% of all space-occupying lesions of the brain cause early epileptic seizures.

3. Nausea with possible vomiting of the "projectile" type.

4. Disk edema. Fundoscopy will reveal a swollen and protruding optic disk with or without hemorrhages. The elevation of the disk can be measured in diopters. The edema is usually more pronounced on the side of the tumor.

5. Focal signs. A tumor of the right hemisphere would affect the left side of the body; this is true for sensory or motor impairment. Speech may be involved if the lesion is on the dominant hemishpere. (Even in 90% of left-handed people the speech center is located in the left hemisphere.)

6. False localizing signs. Due to increased intracranial pressure the abducens nerve may get compressed on the ipsilateral or contralateral side, thus making this sign of little localizing value (see page 7).

7. Lethargy. Drowsiness, sleepiness and slowness of physical and mental reactions will gradually develop. The patient is usually not as alert as before and has difficulty in remembering.

Tests To Be Done

1. Skull X-rays may reveal a shift of the pineal gland which is usually calcified in the adult population. It may also reveal intracranial calcification or erosion of the skull bones.

2. EEG. A slow-wave abnormality (Delta and Theta waves) can be found at and around the site of the tumor. The EEG is not able to differentiate between edema surrounding the tumor and the space-occupying lesion itself. The necrotic part of the tumor is electrically silent.

3. Echoencephalogram may show a displacement of the midline structures away from the space-occupying lesion.

4. Brain scan. Radioactive material is usually taken up in the tumor, especially if the tumor is highly vascularized (glioblastoma).

5. CT-scan of the head is probably the most important non-invasive test which can be done in cases of brain tumors. It will show an increased density in the area of the lesion. Smaller tumors in the brain stem or medulla can be missed by this procedure.

6. Arteriogram. This may reveal shifting of normal cerebral vessels and demonstrate abnormal vessels (arteries) inside or around the tumor. Enlargement of the draining veins may be observed.

Differential Diagnoses

1. Primary Tumors
   a) Neuroepithelial

   i. *Astrocytoma, oligodendroglioma and ependymoma.* These tumors consist of astrocytes, oligodendroglial or ependymal cells, respectively. They are fairly well localized and can generally be removed.

ii. *Glioblastoma*. This tumor, which is the most malignant of all primary brain tumors, involves all of the above cell groups and grows by infiltration. It usually starts on one side and may extend into the corpus callosum and to the opposite hemisphere. Infiltration of the brain substance makes it almost impossible to completely remove. The age of onset is usually between 40–60 years and the survival time generally does not exceed 18 months, although a few cases of survival of 5–10 years have been reported. X-ray radiation and chemotherapy following craniotomy are usually recommended.

b) Mesodermal

Meningioma. This is a relatively benign, well-localized tumor growing from the meninges and can easily be removed if diagnosed early; it does not infiltrate. It is frequently manifested by focal (contralateral) seizures, which may spread in a generalized fashion. It probably originates from the arachnoid membrane and grows very slowly, compressing the underlying brain tissue.

c) Ectodermal

Craniopharyngioma. This type of tumor grows from the lining of the pharynx (Rathke's pouch) and extends into the pituitary fossa and can cause hormonal disturbances.

d) Congenital tumors

These exist and grow from birth on and may have skin, hair or teeth within them. Cutaneous glands may also be found. The tumors are designated as *dermoid* or *epidermoid*.

e) Vascular tumors

These are space-occupying lesions which are a conglomeration of abnormal blood vessels (arteries and veins), which rupture easily, causing pressure usually on the underlying brain. Frequently, focal seizures occur, or rupture of pathological blood vessels may cause a subarachnoid hemorrhage. The diagnosis can usually be made at the age of 10–20 years because during these years the symptoms first appear. Occasionally the skin of the head overlying the brain tumor may show abnormal vascularization.

2. Secondary Tumors

Lesions of this type are usually carcinoma (or sarcoma) metastases which have spread from other sites. They may spread to the brain or spinal cord. The most frequent primary tumors are in the lungs or breast. Cancer of the prostate may metastasize to the bone of the skull and cause pressure upon the underlying brain. These malignant tumors tend to be multiple rather than single and are quite variable in size. Diagnosis is usually made by CT-scan or arteriography. X-ray treatment and chemotherapy are often used. Only in cases of single metastasis is surgical intervention advocated by some neurosurgeons. Life expectancy is generally one and one-half to two years after onset.

B. SPINAL CORD TUMORS

Tumors in this region may cause major symptoms early because of the narrow canal. The most frequent types are *meningioma, lipoma* and *fibroma*. They are benign and do not infiltrate; some, however, may degenerate to malignancy. Metastases from cancer do occur, especially after the age of 50 years, causing severe back pain.

Symptoms

1. Pain radiating into one limb is usually the first sign. The dolor is aggravated when lying flat and thereby stretching the nerve roots. Patients therefore usually have a marked pain at night.

2. Weakness of the limb may develop due to compression of the nerve roots.

3. Reflexes may be diminished or absent in a particular segment.

Tests To Be Done

A spinal tap will show an elevated protein below the lesion (100–200 mg%). By use of a manometer, and manual pressure upon the jugular veins, the spinal fluid will *not* rise rapidly in cases of larger tumors (Queckenstedt's sign). A myelogram will outline the tumor and differentiate between an intramedullary and an extramedullary space-occupying lesion.

All tumors should be operated upon as soon as possible and X-ray radiation can be used after surgical intervention.

Chapter 13

TRAUMA OF THE CENTRAL NERVOUS SYSTEM

Lacerations to the skull or cranium should not be regarded lightly, for they pose the danger of possible spread of infections to the brain, especially in cases of skull fractures and open wounds. Cerebral injuries are therefore of primary concern. The number of cerebral injuries has steadily increased over the past decade, with most being due to motor vehicle accidents. Advances in diagnosis and neurosurgical techniques, however, have lowered the mortality rate in the past few years. The proportion of penetrating wounds of the cranium remains small, except among the military in times of war, and then such lesions increase markedly.

1. Skull Fracture

The danger is that bacteria of different types may get into the cranial cavity and irritate the meninges, which are sterile.

a) *Simple skull fracture.* Diagnosis is usually made by inspection. Occasionally crepitation during palpation at the fracture site is noted; X-rays will confirm the fracture. In cases of hairline fractures no major clinical findings are present. Repeat X-ray studies should be made a few months later to see whether the fracture is healing. The patient is usually put to rest for 5-10 days, after which time he is allowed to ambulate. A careful neurologic examination is done to rule out any injury to the brain.

b) *Compound skull fracture.* This is an injury with major laceration of the scalp, needing stitches. The possibility of infection is great and, therefore, the wound should always be carefully cleansed. Antibiotics may have to be given.

c) *Depressed skull fracture.* In this type of injury the bone is driven into the cranial cavity by a hard blow (hammer, iron bar, etc.). This is considered an emergency and has to be corrected surgically as soon as possible, preferably, within the first few hours. If a piece of bone compresses and irritates the brain cortex the patient may subsequently develop focal epileptic seizures. The bony fragment should be returned surgically to its normal position immediately.

2. Cerebral Concussion

With this type of trauma the patient loses consciousness temporarily when the intracranial pressure is higher than systolic blood pressure. Unconsciousness for a few seconds generally has no serious after-effects. The longer the time of unconsciousness (several minutes or hours), the more likely there will be neurologic sequelae. This result is due to the extensive vibration which has passed through the brain.

Usually no gross anatomical damage is found. Patients with cerebral concussion experience retrograde amnesia and, following the return of consciousness, can not remember events a few seconds or minutes before the accident. Memory is regained slowly (in most cases, up to the time of the accident). An EEG, when taken soon after the accident, may reveal a mild, diffuse cerebral dysrhythmia.

3. Cerebral Contusion

In this injury the patient is unconscious for a longer period of time (several minutes, hours or days) and definite microscopic brain lesions are found. Also, macroscopic evidence of brain involvement is usually seen. For legal purposes, "coup" and "contre-coup" lesions must be separated. The coup is the primary blow to the head and resultant brain injury, and the contre-coup is the secondary cerebral lesion resulting from the head hitting another object.

The brain, which has been accelerated, may be damaged in both instances. Necrotic lesions with diapedetic hemorrhages can be found. The coup and contre-coup lesions are transmitted on the lines of force through the brain substance. A frequent coup lesion is found in the frontal and temporal lobe areas.

In the necrotic region chromatolysis of cells and swelling of fibers occurs; surrounding the focal trauma is brain edema. This may increase for as long as nine or 10 days after the accident and then usually subsides. Later on, due to microglial infiltration, scar formation will start.

The EEG is abnormal and commonly shows a slow-wave focus. Epileptic seizures may result six months to two years later. According to some sources it can take up to 15 years for the post-traumatic seizures to develop. Cerebral contusions are treated in the acute phase with cortisone and diuretic medication. Vital functions should be closely monitored and bed rest is indicated. Close neurosurgical supervision is desirable.

4. Epidural Hematoma

This is bleeding outside the dura mater, usually due to rupture of an artery. The middle meningeal artery is frequently involved because of a fracture of the overlying temporal bone. *These hematomas are an absolute emergency* because of the force and rapidly increasing extent of the bleeding. It is often the cause of death in boxers and football players (the use of helmets is a safeguard). The classical symptoms include head trauma with unconsciousness for a few seconds, followed by headaches.

Twenty to 30 minutes later weakness develops on the opposite side of the body. As the intracranial pressure increases, the patient gradually becomes lethargic and may lose consciousness. The pupil on the side of the hematoma is frequently dilated, while the op-

posite pupil remains normal in size. The patient should be transferred to the hospital as soon as possible. Skull X-rays will demonstrate the fracture line in the temporal bone passing over the
middle meningeal artery.

The patient should be operated on as soon as possible, to
suture the artery before the intracranial pressure becomes excessive. The procedure is not always successful because of the time
factor. Rarely, epidural hematomas occur in the posterior fossa
or from venous hemorrhage. Occasionally, there is enough time
to do a CT-scan or an arteriogram.

5. Subdural Hematoma

This type of bleeding is more benign than epidural hematoma
because venous hemorrhages are not as forceful as arterial. A
subdural hematoma is most likely to occur in young children under
the age of 10 and in older people over the age of 60. Alcoholics
who have a history of frequent falls are predisposed to this complication. Evidence of a blow to the head can usually be found,
although the trauma does not have to be severe in order to rupture
a vein (especially if there is a vitamin K deficiency). Generally,
the older the patient is, the longer it takes for the bleeding to
cause symptoms, since the brain is somewhat smaller at 70-80 years
of age. The pupil on the ipsilateral side is dilated, and a contralateral weakness in the arm and leg develops. The detection of a
subdural hematoma is by CT-scan (revealing a decreased density
in the acute phase and an increased density in the chronic phase)
or by arteriography (revealing the blood vessels not reaching the
inner table of the skull). Usually there is enough time to do these
tests before surgical treatment. Craniotomy to evacuate the ex-
travasated blood is usually necessary.

6. Intracerebral Hematoma

This is a condition frequently occurring in victims of severe motorcycle or automobile accidents. The pupil on the side of the

hemorrhage is dilated due to compression of the oculomotor nerve (III). The opposite side of the body shows weakness in the form of paresis or paralysis. If the hemorrhage is relatively small, the patient can be watched during bed rest in the trauma ICU; a larger hemorrhage may have to be evacuated by craniotomy. The diagnosis is made by CT-scan or arteriography. If the hematoma ruptures into the ventricle the condition of the patient may deteriorate. CT-scan is helpful because it may show blood accumulations in the ventricular system.

7. Fractures Involving the Frontal Sinuses or the Nose

Fracture of the sinuses may cause spinal fluid to drain into the nasal cavities. If the meninges are ruptured, the spinal fluid will drip out of the nostrils. The fluid can be differentiated from the nasal drainage of a common cold by analysis of the contents (especially sugar). The treatment is by neurosurgical intervention in order to avoid infection of the meninges. The patient may have to be placed on antibiotics, because a meningitis can result from migration of nasal contamination (bacteria), and therefore the dura should be sutured quickly.

8. Trauma to the Spinal Cord

Injuries which cause fractures of the vertebrae may result in compression of the spinal cord and the tracts therein. This can be treated with traction and bed rest. *Hematomyelia*, which causes similar symptoms to those of syringomyelia (see page 107), is due to a bleeding into the spinal cord after contusion of the vertebral column. The spinothalamic tracts are interrupted, with loss of pain and temperature sensations. The sensation of touch may be unaffected. If a fracture compresses and interrupts the flow of blood in the *anterior spinal artery*, the patient may lose mainly the pyramidal tract functions below the lesion. If the *posterior spinal arteries* are involved, a marked sensory loss below the lesion may result.

Chapter 14

CONVULSIVE DISORDERS (EPILEPSY)

The word "epilepsy" comes from the Greek and means "to seize upon" or "to overtake." Epileptic seizures have been described since the fifth century BC, and Hippocrates has commented on this brain malfunction. It is more common with inbreeding and is especially prevalent in Peru, Venezuela and Ecuador. The slight preponderance of the disease in males over females is about 13 to 11, and the incidence is higher in the first-born than in the second child and higher in the second child than in the third, and remains about the same in the children which follow. Forty to 50 percent of the people having an epileptiform disorder have convulsions only during the day; 10 to 20 percent have seizures only at night and the remainder have seizures both day and night. Jackson originally described epilepsy as "an occasional, sudden, excessive, rapid and local discharge of the gray matter." The various types are described as follows:

IDIOPATHIC

This entity is, for the most part, congenital, but no definite mode of inheritance is known. A definite family history exists in 35% of epileptics. If one parent has epilepsy the chances of the children having the same disorder are 1 out of 40. With both parents affected the chances are 1 out of 10. The co-twin of identical twins has a 94% chance of having seizures if one twin is affected. It should be understood that epilepsy is actually a syndrome and not a disease. In girls the symptoms usually start with the onset of menstruation (ages 12-14), and in boys also at the time of puberty. This onset may be related to hormonal imbalances and/or water retention in the body and brain, triggering seizures.

SYMPTOMATIC

This type of convulsive disorder is related to other diseases. An inheritance factor is probably present but not definitely established.

1. Trauma

Persons with a family history of epilepsy are probably more likely than those without this history to get post-traumatic seizures after a severe head injury. A *closed injury to the skull* may result in a 5% incidence of post-traumatic seizures. Such a patient usually has been in a coma for several hours or days, and the seizures then appear from six months to two years later. In *penetrating wounds to the brain* the incidence of subsequent seizures is increased to about 15%. (See page 118.)

2. Brain Tumor

Fifteen to 20 percent of patients have a seizure as the first sign of this abnormal growth (see page 111). Later on, approximately 40% of all brain tumors will produce epileptic attacks. Seizures appearing after the age of 25 years should be investigated carefully to rule out a space-occupying lesion.

3. Cerebral Atrophy of Different Etiologies Involving the Cortex

4. Brain Abscess

Seizures usually occur in the acute phase, but also later on due to scar formation.

5. Encephalitis

This is due to inflammation of the gray matter, especially the cortex. Seizures here are regarded as a grave sign.

6. Cerebro-Vascular Disease

Seizures may occur from six months to two years after a stroke in 20% of the cases. Since cerebro-vascular accidents usually involve the white matter, seizures are not as common and generally do not occur within the first few weeks. (See page 41.)

7. Alcohol and Barbiturate Intoxication

This may produce so-called withdrawal seizures, and can occur in other types of drug withdrawal. In cases of barbiturate medication the drug should, therefore, *never be withdrawn abruptly*.

Causes of Symptoms

Pathologic alterations of the cells in the hippocampal area (Sommer sector) are believed to be the after-effects of seizures due to anoxia. Degenerations, leading to reduced numbers of cells, are seen in these regions in most epileptics. Scar tissue may form in the meninges as a result of trauma, brain tumor or abscesses and over a period of time compress the underlying cortex, producing irritation and subsequent seizures. Blood vessels may be compressed by scar tissue, causing hypoxia and secondary epileptic attacks. A focal electrical potential usually occurs in the cortex; in focal seizures the discharge is localized in a certain, well-circumscribed area. If the motor strip on the left side is irritated in the hand region, the right hand will start to shake. If the electrical signal is strong enough it will spread to other parts of the brain, possibly to the opposite hemisphere (by way of the corpus callosum), and a major seizure may occur. The epileptic impulses are carried by the pyramidal tract to the anterior horn cells and from there to the extremities. Everybody is a potential epileptic; the so-called "normal" person has only a slightly higher threshold than the epileptic. Cardiazol injections can produce seizures in almost everyone, as will prolonged photic stimulation. After a seizure, caused by excitation of the cells, the area remains electrically silent for a short time (extinction phenomenon). The possibility that the patient will have another seizure immediately after the first one is therefore reduced. Seizures may possibly originate in the brain stem or spinal cord; the cerebellum is not epileptogenic.

The following abnormalities occur in the area of an epileptic focus during a seizure:

- The cells discharge electrical potentials (up to 800 microvolts).
- The blood flow to the area is increased.
- The oxygen consumption is increased locally and more glucose is needed.
- The only enzyme to be increased focally, as far as we know, is acetylcholinesterase.

The patient may learn to possibly stop a focal seizure by grabbing hold of the shaking extremity (arm or leg). This hold represents a sensory input to the central nervous system, altering the seizure threshold. Seizures can be induced by rapidly inter-rupting light rays by means of the hands (rapid waving in front of the eyes). Patients sometimes do this purposely to aggravate the condition, before being examined, in order to impress the ex-aminer with the seriousness of their condition. Creatine-phos-phokinase (CPK) is increased after a seizure as a result of the rapid contractions of the skeletal musculature. This temporary increase of CPK (which also occurs in strenuous physical exercise such as jogging) must be differentiated from idiopathic muscle disease. (See page 71.)

Tests

1. *Skull film.*   Abnormal calcification in cases of arteriovenous malformations or tumors may occur.

2. *Electroencephalogram.* **(See Fig. 4).** In the waking stage and in sleep. Provocation techniques may have to be used to elicit the seizure phenomenon (hyperventilation, photic and auditory stimulation).

3. *CT-scan.* **(See Fig. 9).** This is done especially if a tumor is suspected. The scan may also show evidence of cerebral atrophy or enlargement of the ventricular system.

4. *Arteriography.* **(See Fig. 7).** Done particularly in cases of tumors or vascular malformations.

Types of Seizures

1. Major (grand mal) seizure. The patient may be able to tell several hours or days ahead of time that a seizure is approaching. This anticipatory sense is called the *prodromal sign*. The patient may experience headache, moodiness or euphoria. These symptoms are not predictable and they vary a great deal, and therefore they are not particularly helpful in localizing the seizure. In the *second stage* an aura or warning may occur. The *aura* is more frequent in longstanding cases and occurs in approximately 50% of epileptics. It is more frequent several years after the onset of the disorder than in the beginning. It is also more common in the higher intellectual group.

The aura is an excellent localization sign for diagnosis. For example: flashing lights would indicate irritation in the occipital cortex, numbness in the left hand would indicate an irritative lesion in the right sensory cortex. A gastric aura (nausea or stomach pressure) indicates temporal lobe origin. A visual aura of an image and an auditory aura of certain sounds may also indicate temporal lobe origin. An aura of smell (usually foul) occurs with a lesion in the uncus of the temporal lobe.

Motor speech is involved if the epileptic focus is located in Broca's area. A patient with a unitemporal lobe focus for 5-10 years may acquire a "mirror focus" in the opposite hemisphere. Multifocal epilepsies usually carry a poorer prognosis.

In the *third stage* the patient may cry out with what is described as a "bird-like" cry. By now he has lost consciousness. During the *fourth stage* (tonic phase) the arms are first in flexion and then in extension (for a few seconds up to two minutes). The diaphragm is arrested and the patient becomes cyanotic. In the *fifth stage* (clonic phase) there is at first a rapid shaking of the body, which gradually slows and subsides. The patient may bite his tongue or lips and he drools from the corners of the mouth. A tongue blade or stick should be placed between his teeth to prevent lacerations of the tongue and oral mucosa. He may be incontinent of urine or stool. This phase may also last from a few seconds up to two minutes. It is important to note that seizures can stop at any of these stages and it is not unusual for a patient to have just an aura and no tonic-clonic convulsions. In the *postictal stage* the patient usually lies motionless, is in a coma and sweats profusely. The pupils are fixed (no light response) and there is a bilateral positive Babinski sign. He gradually comes out of the comatose state, becomes semi-comatose, lethargic and drowsy and usually falls asleep afterwards. Muscular aching is pronounced (lactic acid accumulation in muscle tissue due to the convulsion).

The patient may go from the postictal stage right into an aura again, without completely regaining consciousness, and have another seizure. If this happens two or three times, it is known as *status epilepticus*, which is an *absolute emergency*, for the following reasons:

- There will be prolonged arrest of the diaphragm. This interferes with breathing (oxygenation), and the brain (especially the gray matter) will be rendered hypoxic.
- The body temperature tends to increase.
- The brain will start to swell, due to cerebral edema.
- The pulse rate may rapidly accelerate.
- Usually the comatose state will deepen.

This situation requires all-out measures of treatment or death may ensue. Intravenous injections are usually used to break the cycle of seizures and worsening effects. Valium (10 mg up to 50 mg) can be injected over a period of 2-3 hours. Occasionally, sodium luminal may have to be used (200-300 mg i.v.). Diphenylhydantoin (Dilantin) can be given intravenously. In rare cases where the seizures cannot be controlled, general anesthesia may have to be resorted to.

In the treatment of major seizures, Dilantin and phenobarbital will usually counteract the irritative condition. Dilantin is given in 100 mg doses orally three or four times per day. It is important to check the blood level of Dilantin after the first ten days; the therapeutic level of Dilantin is between 10-20 μg/ml. If the level is lower than this, no anticonvulsive effect can be expected. If the level is above 20 micrograms/ml, toxic symptoms such as nystagmus, ataxia and lethargy may develop. If Dilantin alone does not control major seizures, phenobarbital may have to be added (30 mg. doses three or four times per day, orally). The blood level of phenobarbital should be determined after ten days (therapeutic range: 15-30 μg/ml).

In New York State the patient has to be seizure-free for one year before being allowed to drive a motor vehicle. The patient should also be advised against working in high places (roofs, etc.) because of the danger of falling and self-injury. He should also avoid working with dangerous machinery, and should not swim alone.

2. Minor (petit mal) seizure. These spells usually start at the age of 10-15 years. The patient does not lose consciousness completely. The symptoms are as follows and may last 2-10 seconds.

- Blinking episodes.
- Staring spells.
- Absentmindedness.
- Sudden falls to the floor without losing consciousness (akinetic seizure).
- Brief jerking movements of the arms or legs (myoclonic episodes).

The diagnosis is usually made clinically with the help of the electroencephalogram (Fig. 4). Ninety percent of the cases have abnormal spike and slow waves on the EEG. These discharges usually last a few seconds; they can be triggered by hyperventilation and photic stimulation.

Continuous discharges for days are possible but unusual. During the time of the discharges the patient cannot pay attention and is in a drowsy state. Status epilepticus of minor seizures can occur; 80% of the patients with minor spells will have a major seizure at one time or another. (This usually occurs when the electrical potentials get very strong and spread to other cortical regions.) It is thought that the minor seizures are a result of abnormal cortico-reticular activity.

The treatment of minor seizures consists of ethosuximide (Zarontin) 250 mg three or four times per day, orally. Ten days after inauguration of Zarontin the blood level should be checked (therapeutic range: 30-100 μg/ml). As with major seizures, phenobarbital can also be used (oral dose of 30 mg three or four times per day). Valproic acid (Depakene) should be used if the above two medications are not helpful. The usual dosage of valproic acid is 250 mg 3-4 times per day. The blood level should be checked ten days after inauguration (therapeutic range: 50-100 μg/ml). Because of the side effects, it is necessary to see the patient at regular intervals of 2-3 months and to check the blood for liver and other functions. As a last resort in the treatment of minor seizures, a ketogenic diet (which increases the blood ketones) should be tried. Minor seizures do occur more frequently if the blood sugar level is low, and therefore frequent snacks are recommended and the patient should also be encouraged to eat breakfast each morning.

3. Psychomotor epilepsy (focal seizure with complex symptomatology). These seizures usually occur in adults. Purposeful movements at irrelevant times and places occur. The temporal lobe and posterior part of the frontal lobe are generally involved. The seizures may last from a few seconds to two minutes. In the past, 20% of the patients in psychiatric institutions were known to have this condition. Many patients with schizophrenia and paroxysmal psychiatric episodes should be checked for this particular type of seizure disorder. In these attacks the patient may become destructive and abusive; he may suddenly start to walk out of the room, rub his arm, undress, sing or attack someone. The treatment for psychomotor epilepsy is primidone (Mysoline) (250 mg. orally, three or four times per day). The therapeutic blood levels for Mysoline are 5-12 μg/ml. If Mysoline does not prove effective, Tegretol, which is somewhat more toxic, should be used. The therapeutic blood level is 4-8 μg/ml.

4. Focal epilepsy. This may also occur in cases of trauma and tumor, and focal (sensory or motor) seizures may result. The patient may notice a pinprick feeling (dysesthesia) lasting for a few seconds or minutes affecting one side of the body. He may also notice shaking of one arm and one leg, which might last for hours or days. In Jacksonian epilepsy (which can be of the motor or sensory type), the seizure begins in one part of the body (i.e., the right facial area) and spreads to the right hand and foot. This Jacksonian spread requires only a few seconds. There is usually no loss of consciousness unless the electrical signals are so strong that they spread to other parts of the cortex causing a generalized seizure. (In migraine headache a sensory spread may also take place; this usually takes minutes rather than seconds, however).

Prognosis

Ninety percent of all patients with seizures improve considerably with conservative treatment. If the seizures have been well controlled and the patient suddenly exhibits more frequent attacks, psychological reasons (psychogenesis) should be looked for. It may also be possible that the patient did not take the medication as directed. *Alcoholism* may interfere with the treatment and there is recent evidence that heavy smoking decreases the effect of Dilantin and phenobarbital. Only 0.2% (1 out of 500 patients) require surgical intervention in order to remove the scar causing the epileptic seizures. Craniotomy after an electrocorticogram should be performed to localize the exact primary seizure focus. After a few months or years another epileptic focus may occur near the excised area (due to surgical trauma) and a second surgical procedure may become necessary.

Treatment with antiepileptic drugs should be continued until the patient is free of seizures for at least three to five years. In cases of surgical intervention, the patient should have been treated before with different types of medication for an extensive period of time.

It is important that the patient be employed and has work. Occupational therapy can be of value to these individuals by introducing them to various skills, crafts and hobbies. They should participate in social activities as much as possible. Although epilepsy still carries a stigma, it should be handled in the same manner as any other known disease. This is sometimes not easy because of pronounced egocentricity, irritability and restlessness which can be observed in some of these patients.

TEST QUESTIONS

The "True and False" and "Multiple Choice" questions which follow are typical of those used in neuroscience courses and are presented here as an aid to study. The omission of the answers will require the student to verify his or her choice of answers by consulting the text material. Many students like to prepare for forthcoming tests by studying old examinations when they are available. This technique is a good one but is only of value if the answers are not readily at hand.

A. True or False. (Encircle the appropriate answer.)

1. Multiple sclerosis is most likely to occur after the age of 45 years.   T   F

2. Disk edema, or swelling of the optic disk, is frequently found in patients with multiple sclerosis.   T   F

3. Disk edema is always associated with a marked decrease in vision.   T   F

4. If a patient with symptoms of a brain tumor develops right-sided ataxia, the lesion is most likely in the right cerebellar hemisphere.   T   F

5. If a patient with an intracerebral hemispheric abscess develops right-sided hemiparesis, the lesion is likely to be in the right hemisphere.   T   F

6. In diabetic polyneuropathy the deep tendon reflexes are usually increased.   T   F

7. Dopamine-depletion of the substantia nigra and the pallidum is very frequently found in Parkinson's disease.   T   F

8. Poliomyelitis usually causes (besides a motor weakness) a sensory deficit in the involved extremity.   T   F

9. Intention tremor (in the finger-nose test) is fre-   T   F
    quently observed in patients with Parkinson's dis-
    ease.

10. "Pill rolling tremor" at rest (4–7 cycles/sec) is most   T   F
    noted in cerebellar disease.

11. In myasthenia gravis the muscular weakness is   T   F
    usually more pronounced in the morning after
    sleep.

12. An epidural hematoma is most frequently due to   T   F
    a rupture of the middle meningeal artery after
    fracture of the temporal bone.

13. In myotonia congenita muscle cramping is always   T   F
    associated with muscular atrophy.

14. Encephalitis may cause extrapyramidal tract signs   T   F
    and epileptic seizures.

15. Methyl alcohol intoxication causes optic atrophy   T   F
    and subsequent extrapyramidal symptoms, due to
    a lesion of the putamen.

B. Multiple Choice
(Encircle the appropriate letter. Only one answer is correct.)

1. Maple sugar urine disease is an inborn error of:
    a. Carbohydrate metabolism.
    b. Amino acid metabolism.
    c. Lipid metabolism.
    d. All of the above.
    e. None of the above.

2. Galactosemia is an inborn error of:
    a. Copper metabolism.
    b. Amino acid metabolism.
    c. Lipid metabolism.
    d. All of the above.
    e. None of the above.

3. Tay-Sachs disease (cerebro-macular degeneration) is a disorder of:
    a. Lipid metabolism.
    b. Carbohydrate metabolism.
    c. Amino acid metabolism.
    d. Alcohol metabolism.
    e. Copper metabolism.

4. All of the following entities cause polyneuropathy except:
    a. Lead poisoning.
    b. Alcoholism.
    c. Diabetes mellitus.
    d. Porphyria.
    e. L-Dopa medication.

5. Group A fibers (myelinated), carrying touch and pressure sensation, are 1–20 microns in diameter and have a conduction velocity (meters/sec) of:
    a. 10–20.
    b. 5.
    c. 30–100.
    d. 100–200.
    e. 20.

6. Group B fibers (myelinated) are 3 microns in diameter and have a conduction velocity (meters/sec) of:
    a. 10.
    b. 20.
    c. 30.
    d. 40.
    e. 60–100.

7. If the right trapezius muscle is weak, the lesion is due to involvement of which nerve:
    a. Right hypoglossal.
    b. Right vagus.
    c. Right facial.
    d. Left accessory.
    e. None of the above.

8. If the tongue is partially atrophic and protrudes to the left
    side, the lesion is due to paralysis of which nerve:
    a. Right hypoglossal.
    b. Left hypoglossal.
    c. Right lingual.
    d. Left lingual.
    e. Right glossopharyngeal.

9. The electroencephalogram (EEG) is a helpful test in all of the
    following conditions except:
    a. Encephalitis.
    b. Cerebellar degeneration.
    c. Major seizures.
    d. Minor seizures.
    e. Focal seizures.

10. The electromyogram (EMG), including nerve-conduction
    studies, is most helpful in the following conditon:
    a. Multiple sclerosis.
    b. Parkinson's disease.
    c. Brain tumor.
    d. Neuropathy.
    e. Spinal cord tumor.

11. A child with cerebral palsy is suspected of having hydro-
    cephalus. The most informative test would be:
    a. Cerebral blood flow studies (Doppler).
    b. CT-scan of the head.
    c. Isotope brain scan.
    d. EEG.
    e. Echoencephalogram.

12. A patient (age 63) is suspected of having a brain tumor. The
    test the neurosurgeon would find to be the least valuable in
    localizing the mass would be:
    a. Arteriogram.
    b. CT-scan of the head.
    c. Isotope brain scan.
    d. Spinal fluid analysis.
    e. Skull film.

13. Fasciculations and fibrillations are denervation potentials and can be seen in all of the following conditions except one:
    a. Amyotrophic lateral sclerosis (ALS).
    b. Carpal tunnel syndrome.
    c. Parkinson's disease.
    d. Tarsal tunnel syndrome.
    e. Guillain-Barré syndrome.

14. In myasthenia gravis the lesion is at the level of the:
    a. Anterior horn cell.
    b. Striated muscle.
    c. Posterior root.
    d. Peripheral motor nerve.
    e. Neuromuscular junction.

15. In a patient with unilateral femoral neuropathy the most likely diagnosis is:
    a. Diabetes mellitus.
    b. Cancer metastasis.
    c. Multiple sclerosis.
    d. Chronic alcoholism.
    e. Syringomyelia.

16. Syringomyelia of the cervical cord is most likely due to:
    a. Trauma.
    b. Chronic alcoholism.
    c. Cancer.
    d. Diabetes mellitus.
    e. Probably congenital in persons with malformations.

17. A 55-year-old woman with increasing dementia has moderately severe generalized cortical atrophy of the brain. She is probably suffering from:
    a. Parkinson's disease.
    b. Pick's disease.
    c. Chronic alcoholism.
    d. Alzheimer's disease.
    e. Arterio-venous malformation.

18. Atrophy of the thenar eminence (opponens pollicis muscle)
    indicates a lesion of the following nerve:
    a. Musculocutaneous.
    b. Ulnar.
    c. Radial.
    d. Axillary.
    e. None of the above.

19. A 35-year-old woman has spells of purposeful movements
    over a period of several years at irrelevant times and places.
    The patient suffers from:
    a. Major seizures.
    b. Minor seizures.
    c. Focal seizure with complex symptomatology.
    d. Migraine.
    e. Cerebro-vascular insufficiency.

20. The female patient described above (19) may have to undergo
    all of the following tests except:
    a. Skull films.
    b. Nerve conduction studies.
    c. CT-scan.
    d. EEG.
    e. Echoencephalogram.

21. Continuing with the previous patient, which condition would,
    primarily, have to be ruled out:
    a. Brain tumor.
    b. Multiple sclerosis.
    c. Parkinson's disease.
    d. Myopathy.
    e. Chronic alcoholism.

22. The Babinski sign is abnormal above which age:
    a. 16 Months.
    b. 2 Months.
    c. 4 Months.
    d. 8 Weeks.
    e. At birth.

23. In progressive muscular dystrophy the lesion is probably at the level of:
    a. Neuromuscular junction.
    b. Peripheral nerve fibers.
    c. Individual muscle fibers.
    d. Peripheral sensory fibers.
    e. None of the above.

24. A 58-year-old man complains of mild and persistent double vision of two weeks' duration without history of trauma. Three months before these symptoms, he had left-sided headache and nausea. During the last week before admission to the hospital, dysphasia and a slowly progressing right-sided weakness of the arm and leg developed. The most likely diagnosis is:
    a. Cerebro-vascular accident.
    b. Epidural hematoma.
    c. Multiple sclerosis.
    d. Subdural hematoma.
    e. Brain tumor.

25. A 19-year-old football player gets knocked down after trauma to the head. After several seconds he is able to get up and resume playing. Shortly afterward, however, he complains of severe headache, double vision and a rapidly developing weakness of the right arm and leg. The most likely diagnosis is:
    a. Subdural hematoma.
    b. Cerebral concussion.
    c. Intracerebral embolism.
    d. Epidural hematoma.
    e. Meningitis.

26. A 78-year-old patient with diabetes mellitus and generalized arteriosclerosis develops a relatively sudden paralysis of the right side of the body and becomes unable to speak (expressive aphasia). He is conscious and, upon examination, the spinal fluid is clear. The diagnosis in this case is most likely:
    a. Intracerebral thrombosis.
    b. Brain tumor.
    c. Intracerebral abscess.
    d. Subdural hematoma.
    e. Epidural hematoma.

27. A 60-year-old woman was involved in an automobile accident with resulting minor injury to the head. Over a period of three weeks she developed a gradual paresis of the left side of the body with signs of increased intracranial pressure. The probable diagnosis is:
    a. Epidural hematoma over the right hemisphere.
    b. Cerebral concussion.
    c. Subdural hematoma over the right hemisphere.
    d. Epidural hematoma over the left hemisphere.
    e. Cerebral contusion.

28. In Parkinson's disease all of the following symptoms can be found except:
    a. "Pill rolling tremor" of 5–7 cycles/sec.
    b. Retropulsion.
    c. Bilateral facial paralysis.
    d. Lateral pulsion.
    e. Mask-like face.

29. A patient with amyotrophic lateral sclerosis reveals atrophy and fasciculations of the distal (forearm) musculature. He also reveals spasticity and increased reflexes in both legs with a positive Babinski sign. The lesions of this disease are affecting the:
    a. Spinocerebellar tracts.
    b. Neuromuscular junctions.
    c. Extrapyramidal tract system.
    d. Anterior horn cells and pyramidal tracts.
    e. Anterior horn cells.

30. An 18-year-old girl suffered a severe head injury with prolonged unconsciousness. Eighteen months later she developed short attacks of irrational behavior and occasional major seizures. The probable diagnosis is:
    a. Encephalitis.
    b. Meningitis.
    c. Hysteria.
    d. Post-traumatic amnesia.
    e. Post-traumatic psychomotor epilepsy.

31. A 75-year-old man suffers a thrombotic event of gradual onset involving mainly the proximal part of the left leg and, to a lesser extent, the left arm. The abnormality would involve the following vessel:
    a. Left anterior cerebral artery.
    b. Right anterior cerebral artery.
    c. Left middle cerebral artery.
    d. Right middle cerebral artery.
    e. Vertebro-basilar arterial system.

32. Tuberculous meningitis in a 30-year-old patient, causing severe headaches, slight fever and marked nuchal rigidity, most likely affects the:
    a. Meninges of the convexity of the brain.
    b. Basal ganglia.
    c. Cerebellum.
    d. Meninges of the base of the brain.
    e. White matter of the brain.

33. In a patient with epidural hematoma due to bleeding of the middle meningeal artery after head injury the treatment of choice should be:
    a. Surgical intervention after 2–3 days bed rest.
    b. Surgical intervention after 16–18 hours bed rest.
    c. Surgical intervention immediately (craniotomy).
    d. Administration of tranquilizers.
    e. None of the above.

34. The treatment of polyneuropathy due to chronic alcoholism should definitely include which of the following medications:
    a. Vitamin B_1.
    b. Vitamin B_6.
    c. Vitamin B_{12}.
    d. Aspirin.
    e. Prostigmin.

35. Which of the following is not a warning sign of a stroke in evolution:
    a. Episodes of intermittent weakness of the opposite side of the body.
    b. Episodes of intermittent tingling or numbness of the opposite side of the body.
    c. Intermittent blindness.
    d. Intermittent deafness.
    e. Intermittent speech difficulties.

REFERENCES

Aita, J.A. 1964. Neurologic Manifestations of General Diseases. Charles C Thomas, Springfield.

Barr, M.L. 1972. The Human Nervous System. Harper and Row, New York.

Bodechtel, G. 1958. Differentialdiagnose Neurologischer Krankheitsbilder. Georg Thieme Verlag, Stuttgart.

Carter, S. and Gold, A.P. 1974. Neurology of Infancy and Childhood. Appleton-Century-Crofts, New York.

DeJong, R.N. and Sugar, O. 1978. The Yearbook of Neurology and Neurosurgery. Yearbook Medical Publishers, Inc., Chicago-London.

DeJong, R.N. and Sugar, O. 1979. The Yearbook of Neurology and Neurosurgery. Yearbook Medical Publishers, Inc., Chicago-London.

Ford, F.R. 1966. Diseases of the Nervous System in Infancy, Childhood and Adolescence. 5th edition. Charles C Thomas, Springfield.

Forster, F.M. 1973. Clinical Neurology. 3rd edition. C.V. Mosby, St. Louis.

Gilroy, J. and Meyer, J.S. 1975. Medical Neurology. 2nd edition. The Macmillan Company, New York.

Kiloh, L.G. and Osselton, J.W. 1961. Clinical Electroencephalography. Butterworth Inc., London.

Mayo Clinic and Foundation for Medical Education and Research. 1963. Clinical Examinations in Neurology. W.B. Saunders Company, Philadelphia.

Penry, J.K. 1977. Epilepsy—The Eighth International Symposium. Raven Press, New York.

Plum, F. and Posner, J.B. 1972. Diagnosis of Stupor and Coma. 2nd edition. F.A. Davis Company, Philadelphia.

Schade, J.P. and Ford, D.H. 1965. Basic Neurology. Elsevier Publishing Company, Amsterdam.

Schaltenbrand, G. 1969. Allgemeine Neurologie. Georg Thieme Verlag, Stuttgart.

Scheinberg, P. 1977. Modern Practical Neurology. Raven Press, New York.

Scott, D. 1976. Understanding EEG. J.B. Lippincott Co., Philadelphia.

Smith, B.H. 1965. Principles of Clinical Neurology. Yearbook Medical Publishers, Inc., Chicago.

Smorto, M.D. and Basmajian, J.V. 1972. Clinical Electroneurography. The Williams and Wilkins Company, Baltimore.

Zuelch, K.J. 1965. Brain Tumors, Their Biology and Pathology. 2nd edition. Springer Publishing Company, Inc., New York.

INDEX